Stress Free

One Oh Zee

Jim Schrang

ISBN 0-7414-3033-9

Library of Congress Control Number 2004117558

Published by:

INFINITY PUBLISHING.COM

1094 New DeHaven Street, Suite 100
West Conshohocken, PA 19428-2713
Info@buybooksontheweb.com
www.buybooksontheweb.com
Toll-free (877) BUY BOOK
Local Phone (610) 941-9999
Fax (610) 941-9959

Printed in the United States of America

Printed on Recycled Paper

Published February 2006

Contents

Preface *vi*

ONE The Glory Days 3

TWO EMS What A Mess
The Civilian Gods (EMS Chiefs) 37

THREE Stress Free One Oh Zee 77

FOUR Fidney Paupers *or*
The Twilight of the Gods *121*

FIVE Just Another Day in Paradise *155*

SIX Special Ops, Special
Moments, Special People *211*

Preface

The short, potbellied, anemic EMS officer bolted like a typhoon from behind the cluttered, coffee-stained desk, screaming, "Schrang! You are never going to work overtime again here! I *know* you did this!" His face was fire red, venomously contorted with gigantic jugular veins ready to explode.

"Fuck you, asshole! Prove it," I said, turning into him as he stormed toward me.

Suddenly stopping dead in his tracks, he realized the demented rage would cost him more than his job. Now reduced to only a cold livid glare, fists clenched, he and all present knew he *couldn't prove it*. Turning, I started to walk out of the County office for the last time, when I stopped and looked over my shoulder. There the officer stood, frozen in time, shoulders hunched forward, ego deflated, fists still clenched. I smiled, watching him tremble with untold hatred, before continuing toward my car. Soon my little red Honda was flying along the empty Interborough Parkway. Looking up the hill to my right toward Rene's plot, I noticed how crowded the cemetery had become. I thought of what the captain had tried to pin on me. Talk about a battle of wits. Hell, this guy was totally unarmed. We had responded to a cardiac arrest. My partner, I and the EMTs worked hard to get the patient's pulse and blood pressure back. Having succeeded, we brought the now viable patient to the infamous Brooklyn Hospital. The emergency room staff didn't have a stretcher or a clue, so they continued to work the patient on our stretcher. Then, an idiot doctor pushed the wrong drug, killing the patient instantly, this time for good. Such a mistake was not, is not, uncommon.

"What the fuck did you just do, doc?" I asked in a very tired, weary voice.

"Do not worry! Show respect, I am a doctor, you know!"

"You're an asshole!" I yelled, lunging across the stretcher as he ran from the room.

"Jim! Fuck him, let's go home," my partner said, trying to calm me down after seeing this third-world urchin outright kill our patient, and knowing nothing would ever come of it because of the M.D. title.

The only other problem was that the dead patient was on *our* stretcher. Yeah, I know paramedics always use the EMT's stretcher, but they had tickets for a Yankee game and needed to get off on time. So we did our good deed, and you know what that means in NYC EMS land: "No good deed will not go unpunished." Now that the useless staff couldn't come up with a stretcher, I called for a patrol supervisor. His job was to expedite such matters. Once on the scene, he told me not to worry, "You're on overtime, so pull up a chair and relax."

"Look, I'm tired and just want to get out of here," I replied, my shirt and pants reeking from sweat as the patrol boss told my partner to get a chair. I had a chair, the patient had our stretcher, my partner went to restock and the "boss" went on his merry way. A little while later, I came out with our stretcher, placed it in the ambulance, and we went to Kings County for a change of tour.

Once we got there, the captain asked, "What did you guys do?"

"Don't know what you mean. Good night," I said grabbing the narcotic and sign-out logs.

"Schrang!" he exploded. "You are never going to work overtime again here! I *know* you did this!"

"Did what?" my partner asked, looking totally confused as he signed in the narcotics. Several crewmembers were now standing by the door, listening.

"Where did you leave the patient?"

"In the hospital."

"*Where* in the hospital?"

"In the ER, on a stretcher."

"No, you didn't!" he shouted.

"What the fuck are you talking about?" my partner asked.

"I received a call from the administrator who said a Filipino nurse walked into the nurses' lounge and found the deceased wrapped in a sheet, with the intubation tube still in his mouth along with a cigarette, holding a coffee cup, legs crossed, sitting in . . . a chair!"

"And your point is?" I asked over the howls of laughter from my partner and crews standing by.

"She screamed, passed out, hitting her head so badly, it took thirteen stitches to close the wound!"

"Gee, sucks to be her, huh? The hospital is not on my list of best-known facilities for medical care, and smoking *is* bad for your health."

As I drove toward Queens, the warm air felt good as the smell of the flowers from the park enraptured me. A full moon was coming up. Suddenly the magic was worked. I was no longer upset that someone would even suggest *maw* would do such a thing. Hell, I don't even smoke. Suddenly I was laughing so hard thinking of the sight that tears filled my eyes.

Stress Free One Oh Zee

ONE

The Glory Days

Great spirits have always encountered violent opposition from mediocre minds. Many of these profound teachers were considered troublemakers.

—ALBERT EINSTEIN, *Wisdom of the Ages*

In 1983, I went on my first ambulance call in Queens, New York with my brother, Tim.

He and another paramedic manned the unit. From that day on, I wanted to be part of the Emergency Medical Service (EMS) of New York City. In November 1983, I said a fond farewell to New York City's Housing Elevator Division to attend the EMS Academy. At that time it was located in several rooms on the sprawling grounds of Queens General Hospital in Jamaica, New York.

These are the stories you never learn about. The depravity, brutality, and love EMS crews experience daily. But it is also an unfiltered, shocking, and sometimes humorous examination of the darkest side of the human condition.

Prior to getting into the academy, I had to pass an EVOC (Emergency Vehicle Operators Course) at Floyd Bennett Air Field in Brooklyn. It was one of those overcast winter days, when the cold winds swept in from Jamaica Bay. We huddled together for warmth. Each candidate wore a pin or a jacket or something from his or her volunteer ambulance core or voluntary hospital. I wore my blue baseball hat from Long Island College Hospital with its EMS logo.

The instructors left their warm trailer to explain the test. First, we had to maneuver through the designated obstacle course. If we knocked over too many plastic cones, did not complete the run in the specified time, lost control, or killed an instructor, we lost points and possibly failed. Upon successful completion of the obstacle course, we had to pass a road test.

I was in line, trying to keep warm, when a man dressed in civilian attire came up and yelled, "Get that hat off. You are not a member of EMS."

I played the game and took off the hat, wondering who this idiot was and why he had singled me out. After the little twerp left, an instructor asked if I knew the guy. I answered no and was told to not let his remarks upset me. He was the head of the personnel department and was intimidating me for some reason.

Finally, it was my turn to take the test. My instructor was Pat Scaringello. Funny, my grandfather's name was Scaringello, prior to changing it to Schrango; the "o" was lost during his service in World War II with the U.S. Navy's famed Construction Battalion (CBs) or Seabees.

A stocky man, Pat was former navy. He and I hit it off when he learned I was a Vietnam veteran and had served in combat as a paratrooper with the 101st Airborne Division, Screaming Eagles.

All the instructors were helpful, knowledgeable, and courteous. They pointed out little things of importance, such as how to adjust the mirrors to see only the white tips of the cones. Such hints helped a lot.

The instructors were our cheerleaders. They wanted us to succeed. If we failed, it was us, not them, who failed. Pat made me feel like a partner, not an inept trainee. I knew I wanted to be a part of this team after meeting these instructors.

The program made good management sense. It weeded out the people who could not cut the driving course, so as not to waste resources of the EMS Academy.

Things got interesting when I reported to the academy. After being in combat, I thought the academy's paramilitary environment was total bullshit. But I played the game. Our uniforms were green pants and ties, white shirts, and softball hats.

Robert Becker, Chief of Operations, ruled by fear. I first saw him when he spoke to our class. We were called to attention, as a rather short, young, brooding male walked into the classroom wearing a dress, green uniform with jacket. He had more ribbons on his jacket than a Russian general. His mannerisms evoked fear in those who were impressed by him, and they responded to his every anticipated need. Everyone stood at attention, except for me. I was at semi-attention, getting a charge out of this wannabe.

Becker was introduced to the class. As he approached the podium, he turned off his radio. I guess it was meant to impress people and make them think he was in control, knowing all, monitoring everything—very important, right?

I saw the fear and unspoken loathing the instructors had for him. His staff was handpicked and catered to his every directive. Standing there like the rest of the candidates, I made mental notes.

After his spiritless speech, he extended his hand and an officer gave him his radio. He turned toward the door, flipped on his radio, and strutted out with his wimpy staff trailing behind. *How awe inspiring.* This was my first taste of EMS leadership.

One day, I was called from class to speak with a young lady. "Someone wants to get you fired." She said that on my application, I had answered "no" to the question about having family on the job. I had an uncle, Chief Robert Regan, but not having seen him since I was twelve years old, he didn't rate. Besides, my career would be built by me, on my own, without family help.

I asked who was out to get me fired. She wouldn't disclose his name but said he was a big cheese in the organization. I mentioned my uncle's name. She revealed that the personnel department administrator, Arnold Pack, and my uncle were good buddies. They were out to get me.

My brother and my uncle had bad blood between them. I only had one confrontation with my uncle. At my mother's funeral, he and his brother made fools of themselves. His brother made a crack about my unit in Vietnam. One word led to another. The chief joined in. Both were former marines, but neither had combat experience. I told them I'd be more than happy to kick their asses. Neither one was stupid enough to come up the stairs to confront me.

I had forgotten the whole episode, but it was evident the chief hadn't and his little rat was watching. I was starting to see how the chain of command actually worked, as she filled me in.

I thanked this angel for giving me a heads up on the situation. That same day, I sent Chief Robert Becker a box filled with medals and citations I'd won in combat. In the accompanying letter, I pointed out there was a major problem in the EMS chain of command. One of his chiefs was not judging candidates by merit, but on personal whim.

A week later I was ordered to report to headquarters in Maspeth, Queens and pick up my decorations. I graduated. To his credit, years later my uncle commended me on the reputation I forged working the streets. He was proud of me. It meant a lot to me then and still does.

While going through the EMS training, I quarried opinions about the worst area to work. I wanted to be in a high-volume area, figuring this would be the optimal environment to learn, and remain out of my uncle's Bronx Command, so I could establish a reputation on my own actions.

King's County in Brooklyn won, without a doubt, the award of being the very worst, most dangerous place in New York City. When the request forms were handed out for assignments every space of my "dream sheet" was filled in with King's County, Brooklyn.

Reporting to King's County garage, I began my career at Station Thirty-three. At thirty-five years old, having survived combat and the tragic death of my wife, I knew I'd adjust to the job. On the rotations, I kept my mouth shut, unlike my other classmates who had cocky know-it-all attitudes. These attitudes caused problems. I was soon assigned a regular time slot and unit.

God, how I loved my job! Being an EMT and working at King's County Hospital was the greatest job in the world and I never wanted to leave it.

Going to work, I drove along the high-speed Grand Central Parkway, cutting across Queens, and entered the Interborough Parkway. The Interborough meandered through lush Forest Hills Park. The majestic trees with their fragrance of the flowers enveloped my car as I approached Dead Man's Curve. Cypress Hills Cemetery loomed to my left side up on high ground. Scattered tombs, statues, and headstones dotted the almost barren hillside, these cold, man-made, solid concrete and marble structures harshly clawed into a soft royal blue sky reminding me of life's frailty.

Passing the Ridgewood Reservoir, I saw kids at play and soon the car started a downward dive in more ways than one. I could feel a distinct change in the atmosphere. Upon leaving the Interborough, emptying onto the three-way merger of Jamaica, Bushwick, and Pennsylvania Avenues in Brooklyn, I could sense the tension, hostility, and excitement in the air.

On the way to King's County, I passed the Pennsylvania Outpost, which made the police department's infamous Fort Apache in the South Bronx look like a Girl Scout camp. It was an outpost surrounded by a sea of trash, broken lives, and utter devastation.

Nearly finishing my route, I drove along Eastern Parkway, where some of the most exquisite buildings of a bygone era stood in various stages of decay. The sense of hopelessness permeated the area like the plague. Yet, if I looked beyond the surface, I could sense the strength, resourcefulness, and hope of this community.

I turned onto Utica Avenue, a highly congested artery. The area was populated with Afro-Americans, including families from the Caribbean Islands and Africa. Pockets of Hasidic Jewish families surrounded the Lubavitch World Headquarters located on Eastern Parkway. This section, known as Crown Heights, was vibrant and colorful. I made the last turn into the County garage.

Stepping out, I said a silent prayer not to screw up. It was here I met Lieutenants Joeddy Friszell and B.J. Flanders. They would become my immediate supervisors and good friends.

Lieutenant Friszell ran the garage by the book—the book he wrote using his army background. He was mission oriented, but worked *with* his people. He did have one minor weakness that nailed him more than once. He tried to take on a paramedic or two in a discussion. He was an EMT.

One day, he went after two medics whose boots weren't spit-shined. "And what's your excuse for not having your boots polished?" he asked the two medics.

They became serious. "Gee, sir, didn't you read the article in the *New England Journal of Medicine*, about the study concerning polishing boots?" one asked.

"No. What did it say?" he asked, now very interested.

"Well, the study said that those who continually spit-shine their shoes and boots eventually go bald."

The lieutenant turned beet red, yelling, "Get out of here!"

Lieutenant Joeddy Friszell was just about bald. He learned fast not to mess with paramedics. Observing these antics, I knew I had the makings of a paramedic. These guys were always up to something to make people laugh. Never let it be said that Lieutenant Joeddy Friszell would remain down after such an invigorating dissertation by such astute paramedics. If he could not convince the medics of his wisdom, he would lead them by example.

Joe spent his own money on a standup, plug-in, shoe polisher for the station. He placed a sign on it, "Now there is *no reason* not to shine your boots." Several days later, Joe returned to the station to find his beloved shoe-polishing machine a tangled, broken pile of scrap metal. He thought an ambulance had accidentally run over it. Accidents do happen. Then he saw the sign in bold black letters. "Now there is *no reason to shine our boots*."

One night, Lieutenant B.J. Flanders caught us out of our area. It was 1:00 A.M. as he yelled at us from his command vehicle. An elderly, homeless woman came between the two vehicles and asked for change. Her hair was matted down, clothes filthy and a stench so putrid it was like the polluted sludge of Flushing River during low tide. I stepped out as Lieutenant Flanders directed his attention to my partner, Joe Sarro.

Stealthily, I walked the old lady to the passenger side of the lieutenant's vehicle, giving her two dollars, signaling her to be quiet as I gingerly opened the door, strapped her in, and gently closed and locked the door. I quickly walked around, got into my vehicle and told Joe, who was holding a straight face, "Let's get out of here."

We took off fast, surprising the good Lieutenant Flanders, who started to say something about a smell. Suddenly our radio came alive with the lieutenant's unprofessional threat.

I had a future here. Joe and B.J. were hardworking, hard-playing men and real leaders. They were always the first to ask if we were all right. The caliber of these men was missing in the micro-managing, paper-pushing world of the EMS gods.

My partner's mom was a police officer in a Brooklyn precinct. Our unit was 32 Adam, or, as I named it, 32 America. The white unit sported an orange stripe with the Health and Hospital logo on the side. On each door was a half-moon EMS logo we placed on an angle. This represented our belief that EMS administration, led by Robert Becker, was not on the level. We taped on American flags; bold letters placed on our doors had our unit designation, 32 America.

We had a blast driving through the streets of Brooklyn, being the first on the scene of a bad MVA (motor vehicle accident), shooting, or heart attack. Sometimes we'd blast the *Star Wars* theme over the PA system as we flew to a job. We built a good reputation, even with the dispatchers.

One day we responded to an "Elderly Sick," whom we found seated alone in her apartment. We were only EMTs but knew this old lady needed paramedics, so I called the board dispatcher. There were a number of units requesting medics and I heard the floor lieutenant tell the dispatcher, "If Thirty-two America is asking, then get them medics." We worked as a team, putting oxygen on the patient, getting vital signs, and making a fast grab at any and all of her medications within arm's reach. Once completed, we started to package the patient by lifting the old lady and strapping her into our collapsible stair chair. We would meet the medics downstairs, or if they weren't there, start moving to the King's County.

As Joe finished the strapping and I did a fast final survey collecting our equipment, in walked two legends from King's County, paramedics William Simon and Sandy Edmondson. At that moment she took a labored breath and went into arrest. We unstrapped then placed her on the floor. Sandy gave her a pericardial thump in her breastbone. The idea was to create enough of an electrical impulse to bring the heart back into a synchronized beating pattern.

I did compressions, while Joe used the BVM (Bag Valve Mask) to breathe for the woman until Sandy intubated her. One of the sickest sounds you will ever hear is when doing compressions on an elderly patient and a rib or two cracks. This was my first experience. As I went down with the compression I heard and felt the crack. Billy looked up from pushing the drugs through the IV and told me, "Don't worry. Just keep doing the compressions."

Later we transported her to King's County where doctors worked on her before moving her upstairs.

As Joe and I were cleaning up our vehicle, Sandy came out and thanked us for our help. He told us we did a great job at realizing the old lady was going out of the picture. In those days, unlike too many of the new breed of EMTs, we took pride in our diagnoses. This was how we learned and built our reputation with the medics. We never asked for medics before we evaluated the patient, thereby developing a sixth sense. Joe and I went back into service. I saw Billy a week later and learned our patient had died.

The weather at the beginning of the tour was warm, but now after the arrest with our shirts wringing wet, it seemed even hotter. We decided to grab a sandwich and soda at a bodega place reportedly owned by the brother of a Coney Island paramedic, Mitch Stern. Stern was one of "Beckers Peckers," earning the nickname by his continuous accolades he would throw concerning Chief Becker. Next we headed to our favorite location on Coney Island Avenue, where a new disco had opened, enjoying the spot because we could check out the girls. What more could we ask for? We new guys had just helped a patient, had been praised by two respected medics, and had good sandwiches. They should have been good, we paid full price. Now we could check out the girls.

A short, plump gold-skinned man approached the vehicle on my side. My window was open and the vehicle was off as we ate. EMS didn't care if the air conditioning worked in the crew section, so long as the patient's compartment worked. This tradition of not caring about the crews continues today. Traditions are important.

At my window, he yelled, "Get this shit ambulance out of here now!"

"What seems to be your problem?" I asked, taking another bite from my sandwich.

"This is *my* club and I don't want you *assholes* parking here."

"Hey, you're the asshole with that poor excuse of a wig, so fuck off," Joe said, as I laughed, almost choking on my sandwich.

The guy spun around with his wig following. "You two guys better not be here next Saturday or you'll get your asses kicked."

"Yeah, yeah, make sure you get some paste for that rug of yours first, asshole," I said.

Shortly before we finished our meal, a frantic 10-13 blared across the radio from one of our units. Signal 10-85 means "I'm about to get my ass kicked," and 10-13 means "I am getting my ass kicked."

The unit was on President Street, treating a male black who had been stabbed. As both crew members worked on the patient, the perpetrator came back.

Just as one of the EMTs was exiting the side door, the perp pushed his way into the back of the vehicle and started shooting erratically, trying to kill the patient. Both crewmembers were trapped in the back of the unit. They tried to hide behind the captain's chair and screamed for assistance. Shots rang out over the radio. When we arrived, we found both crewmembers shaken. Another unit transported the victim.

The perp was still on the loose. One of our bosses arrived, so we took one last look at the situation and went back on patrol.

Our next assignment was an EDP (Extremely Disturbed Person). The police sector car pulled up when we did. We cautiously approached the apartment door. The EMTs were on one side of the door and the cops on the other. One of the cops rapped on the door with his nightstick. The door opened and a female asked us to come in, leading us to the kitchen without so much as a word.

Upon entering, we saw a sixty-year-old black female standing naked, mumbling, "I came into this world naked and I'm leaving the same way."

The younger woman identified herself as the daughter. We wrapped a sheet around the old lady, secured her in the chair, and took her to King's County.

Several calls later, we returned to King's County. We spoke with Lieutenant Bob Moron, a no-nonsense officer and former marine. We told him about the problems with the man at our parking location. He agreed we could park there and, being EMS, we could rest assured no one was going to push us around. He said he'd listen to the radio next Saturday and be ready to respond with baseball bat if we had trouble. Then we said goodnight.

As you may already suspect, the following Saturday as we stopped off for our dinner, we were told, "You guys are in major trouble. The owner of the club came in and asked questions about you two."

"Yeah, and . . . ?"

"He knows I work for EMS and don't want problems, unlike you two. He said to tell you guys that if you cherish your lives, you won't go there again and piss him off."

I told this less-than-adventurous loser, "Well, he just pissed off my partner and me. No one messes with Thirty-two America."

We paid for our meal and pulled up to our parking spot. It didn't take long for the wannabe Guido to come out with a few friends. He walked to my side of the bus (the term for an ambulance in New York City) and started screaming across me, looking at Joey.

"I told you assholes not to park here!"

"Hey, first, knock off the screaming. Next, if you want to talk to my partner, walk around the ambulance to his window," I said.

"I warned you. Now you two assholes are going to get your legs broken."

"Hey," I laughed, "you've been watching too many of those spaghetti westerns." Without taking my eyes off him, I continued. "You're not even a real Italian, probably only Sicilian, an imitation Italian, unlike me. Listen Guido, you're lucky my partner is driving. Otherwise, I'd put the unit right through your glass windows onto the fuckin' dance floor and give new meaning to a disco light show."

So far, Joe was doing well. As long as we were in the vehicle and he was mouthing off outside, who cared? But all good things come to an end.

"That's it. You two are dead."

Joe lost it and shrieked at the guy. "All right, asshole, let's see what you've got!" jumping from the vehicle.

The clown and his four goons moved toward the other side of the bus. One guy looked like the front of the New York Jets, with a face only a mother could ever love. Seeing a gun in his waistband and having my radio in hand I knew I had to even the score fast! I'd use the radio to take down the idiot with the weapon. As I exited the vehicle, I hit two of the idiots with the door and called, "Thirty-two America, ten-thirteen, ten-thirteen!"

Suddenly all hell broke loose on Coney Island Avenue, as I came to stand shoulder to shoulder with Joe. EMS buses from King's County and police cars came flying out of nowhere. Coney Island Avenue became a sea of wailing sirens and flashing red and white lights. So far it was only a shoving match and Guido was losing against a sea of EMS crews and police officers. I tried to get the guy with the weapon as he ran into the disco, so I stayed with my partner and told the sergeant what had happened. The disco lost its cabaret license, was closed, and summoned for the next two weeks. Seemed the disco was on the PD's shit list and now it was on ours.

On the third Saturday, Joe and I stopped for dinner, paid, and parked. Over the radio we were asked to call our station. In those days there were no cell phones and no phones on the corner.

"Gee, there's only one place I see with a phone," I said as I gazed at the disco.

"No! You're crazy," Joe said.

"Trust me," I said with a smile.

"I'll come in with you."

"No, you won't. I'll need you here to come in and pick me up if I have a problem. I'll meet you on the dance floor."

Joe smiled and started the vehicle. I walked into the place and spotted a phone as I was walking past Guido's office! Both he and his clown with the weapon looked up in total shock.

"Hi there," I said as I waved and walked to the phone, dropping in the money. Lieutenant Moron picked up the phone and asked if we were okay.

"Oh, we're fine," I assured him. He asked where I was calling from and I told him, "Inside the disco."

"Where?"

"Inside the disco."

"Are you crazy?"

I looked at the two individuals who were now giving me cold stares. I smiled at them and spoke into the phone, "Hey boss, trust me, we're doing great here. Talk later."

I hung up, smiled, and walked out. Outside, I breathed a sigh of relief. No one pushes EMS around, especially 32 America. Joe and I agreed that since we had neutralized the threat to 32 America, upheld the honor of EMS, it was time to move on. Besides we really didn't enjoy the sandwiches or hospitality anymore.

The amount of pure, unadulterated hatred and fear in East New York during these years was unbelievable. The hatred was manifested in violence, which kept a community in the chains of insane bondage. I was disgusted by the carnage—the broken, mutilated, sometimes lifeless bodies within the black population. Usually, it was black against black, but every now and then the violence would spill over and hit an unsuspecting white. Just as no one culture has the market on ignorance, insanity knows no boundary.

Such was the case one sweltering summer night. A white, non-street-smart, arrogant doctor who worked with disdain on our patients left late from King's County, heading home. Anyone with a grain of common sense, never mind street smarts, knew, after the sun goes down, to lock the car doors and keep the music to a minimum so as not to draw attention. Never stop at red lights or stop signs. Instead, slow down to look both ways, but keep moving, rolling stops. Never pull in behind a car stopped. Instead, leave a distance to pull out fast if someone tries to block you in.

That evening we were hanging outside the ER, talking when a new, white Mercedes came flying up the ramp and screeching to a halt, almost hitting a parked ambulance. We rushed over to find the driver crying hysterically and bleeding from his head.

"Get me out of here! Get me out of here! I'm a doctor," he screamed, like a stuck pig. One of the crew lifted him and he screamed in pain, as his head fell back in agony. He grabbed his left arm. I could see it had been stabbed and broken. As the crew attempted to carry him to the stretcher, he regained his composure.

"I'm Doctor So and So and I'll have your jobs for the way you bastards are treating me!"

At that point he was about three feet above the stretcher when the crew in unison said, "Oops," and he crashed back down on the stretcher, emitting another bloodcurdling scream.

"Do you want to take the piece of shit inside?"

"No, you do it."

"No, we lifted him out."

Through the tears we heard, "For Christ's sake, please get me inside. I'm going to die!"

"Oh shit, all right. We'll take him in." Two other EMTs grabbed the stretcher, bouncing it upon the ramp. They wheeled him into the crash room as we followed where the medical staff recognized him and started their evaluation.

As the nurses started to strip him for the examination he hollered, "Don't let them strip me. I'm Doctor So and So. I'm a doctor!"

The helpful crew members left the patient in the capable hands of the ER staff and returned outside to inspect the damage to the car. We learned later the doctor had the radio blasting as he stopped at a light. Several black males had come up to him and demanded money. He responded to them in his typical self-centered fashion and the thugs responded in theirs. He was punched in the face, stabbed in the arm, and a cinder block was put through his front windshield. As they tried to pull him from the car, his arm was broken, but he managed to speed away.

We never did see that doctor at the hospital again. Sure hope his bedside manners improved.

One night, a crew asked for "extra hands" to offload a patient. They brought in a female patient with something still attached to her vagina. The crew, us, as well as the police officers, gingerly removed the stretcher and cleared the hall, keeping the patient and the large dog, still attached to her, very calm. Yes, her dog was still attached. Once she was inside the exam room, the nurses paged the doctors, including the patient's own husband. This gave a new meaning to "pet lover."

That episode was not anything out of the ordinary. One night, Barry Travis and I responded to an "Injury," according to a laughing dispatcher named Mickie Kave. As we pulled up, we saw two cops, one standing, the other sitting, on the hood of their car laughing. They were rapping with two young, scantily clad, good-looking black females.

"Hey guys, what's so funny?"

"Oh, you'll find out. He's in apartment 1C."

There was an uproar of laughter. Walking in, we found several black males huddled around another, who was holding a towel on his genital area. We asked what was wrong and he opened the towel to show us a torn, bleeding penis. We walked to the bus in silence, with the patient clutching the towel. In his Haitian accent he told how upon entering the super's apartment he had the dog lick his penis. For some unknown reason, the dog chomped down.

As Barry stepped into the back of the bus with the patient, I jokingly asked him, "Hey, are you going to splint it?" Barry laughed heartily as I closed the door.

When we contacted Mickie on the radio, she asked where we were going with the patient. I knew she was curious about the injury, so I said, "We are taking him over to King's County to act as a lawn sprinkler." She couldn't stop laughing.

Barry Travis and I made an interesting team, despite the fact that we didn't like each other when we first met. At King's County, we had an officer or two who weren't of the same cut as Lieutenants Friszell, Flanders, or Moron. There was one officer called Hawk Eye because his eye looked outward instead of in unison with the other eye. Hawk Eye did not like Barry or me. Realizing that we didn't get along, he put us together, figuring we would have a fistfight, he could do the charge package and get us both fired.

To his credit, Barry had a different idea. We became friends and a team, much to the dismay of Hawk Eye.

One day, at King's County, we brought in an ambulance with problem brakes. Hawk Eye was behind the desk and we asked him to put the unit out until roadside repair could check it out. In those days, as today, the guy behind the desk was more concerned with keeping a unit in service than with crew safety. Thus, we were told to stay in the vehicle.

Down the street from King's County was a large, old oak tree. We put across the radio that we didn't feel safe in the vehicle, but the lieutenant ordered us back on the road. We thought it would be a shame, if by chance, as we left the garage, the brakes failed and we crashed into that old tree. Oh what a commotion that would cause.

Hawk Eye aimed towards captain's bars. He wanted us to chase unemployment checks. As we started out of the station, Hawk Eye said he wanted us to transport a sick EMT to the Pennsylvania Outpost.

The pencil-thin, black curly-haired Italian new EMT came up to the unit, demanding, "I'm Jonathan. How long is it going to take to get me back to the Outpost?"

"If I was you, I'd take a city bus, because we are having problems here and we do not plan on moving fast for safety reasons," Barry said. I could attest to EMS's unconcern, since I had a unit where the steering wheel came off in my hands and they did not want to put it out of service! We had ambulances burning, literally going up in flames, on the streets. During the eighties, Lynn Schulman, in Public Affairs, told the press that the units were breaking down "because the crews were sabotaging them, so they did not have to work." She and her statement were sanctioned by Chief Becker.

So we left King's County using due regard for safety as we drove to the Outpost. I pulled into the garage to let out the sick EMT. The side door flew open and the little twerp shrieked, "What took you guys so long? You should be accepting a job by now!"

Barry and I looked at each other. Another avalanche of vulgarity came from the twerp's mouth.

"Enough!" I said as we *got out to put out* somebody's lights.

Several EMTs and medics ran over, yelling, "He's sick. Don't hit him!"

"Then let the little ass wipe plead insanity," I said as Barry reached for him.

The sick, spineless loudmouth ran inside the office and locked the door. We wished everyone a fond adieu and left.

The next day, walking into the garage, I heard Hawk Eye yelling at Barry. He saw me. "Get your ass in here!"

"What did you do last night?" Hawk Eye demanded.

"At what time?" he asked, with a grin.

"I want a written statement of what happened last night after you were ordered to take the sick EMT to the Outpost."

"Okay, no problem."

The written statement said, "Using due regard in a dangerous vehicle, we were ordered to drive against our better judgment; we transported a sick EMT to the Outpost. After dropping him off, we went into service." My partner witnessed it and handed it to Hawk Eye to read.

"What is this shit?" he yelled, as he tore the paper up in a fit of rage. "I know what took place and you two better own up to it."

"Enough," I yelled. "First, when you talk to a man you look him straight in the eyes or don't talk to him!" With this, Barry became hysterical. "Second, if you know something, then put it in writing so we can sue you and EMS."

Hawk Eye recovered from the initial onslaught and attempted to speak. But I was on the offensive and would not yield ground. "Third, it smells like shit in here and I'm not making reference to that stray dog we adopted, so let's get out of here." We both walked out, leaving a dumbfounded Hawk Eye.

But the fun was just beginning for the good lieutenant. As I reached in for a portable oxygen bottle, I pulled my shoulder.

"Oh gee, I hurt my shoulder," I said to Barry.

"I saw that. I'll tell Hawk Eye you need a compensation package." Barry returned, saying with a twinkle in his eye, "He is refusing to give you the package."

"Okay, watch this." I walked in. "Sir, first you accuse us of something with no information to back it up. Next, you're refusing to give me a compensation package. Is this correct?"

"Get out of here. You're not hurt. I know."

"When will you ever learn?" were my final words, as I walked out.

At home, I called the tour commander, who was initially upset about not having the unit run. But the tour commander exploded when he was told that I was refused a compensation package and was thinking of suing all concerned. He was being very apologetic to the good EMT me, and tore a chunk from the ass of the bad lieutenant.

Two days later, I healed and returned to work. I discovered that Hawk Eye had received a phone call. The transported sick EMT called Hawk Eye, saying that his life was threatened, not by one, but both of us EMTs. Nothing was ever verified. Even the crews at his own station could not stomach this ass wipe. This sick EMT, aside from being spineless, became a lieutenant in one of the borough offices, or as we called them, the Enchanted Forest, and "Puzzle Palace" to Location One, Headquarters in Maspeth, Queens.

As the temperature increased, the senseless violence spiraled in East New York. People were getting shot and butchered at an unbelievable rate. We called ourselves County Mounties, a no-nonsense, hard-playing group of people. In those days, if you had a problem with a partner, you spoke. If that didn't work, you'd use old-fashioned methods. More than one crew walked into the ER, having "fallen off the back of the bus." When it was over, both crew members would have a beer.

There was a silent code of family that no one outside EMS could threaten or hurt a co-worker. The cops and perps had guns. We had to develop street smarts to survive, or as I called it, officer presence. Often we would be the first to enter a crack house for an"injury," which was actually a violent family dispute with an injury. In the ghetto, respect was everything, the common denominator not only to helping people but, more importantly, surviving, period. Stepping into totally hostile environment, outnumbered, unarmed, you had to learn to take charge of the situation first. This meant not taking shit from anyone, weapon or not. If you blinked, you lost respect, the result being you placed your partner and your life in danger. Sometimes it took a little physical adjustment of the people's attitude to have them realize we, not they, were in charge. I told a rowdy patient, "Listen, we are here to help you. After work we are either going home or to work overtime. But understand if anyone is going to get hurt, it will not be my partner or me." He got the point and cooperated. Once we established the respect, it became now a matter of diffusing the original situation by dividing up the combatants, sometimes into different rooms. This took a lot of unspoken trust between partners. Finally, we needed them to work together for the common good of the patient on whom we could now focus. They might have the guns, but we weren't the little white boys who came in from Long Island to buy drugs. We were the ghetto EMTs and paramedics who were the psycho healers. We could drown you in compassion and perhaps treat you with the first honest, loving concern you had in your life or we could kick your fuckin' ass and you'd die, literally. In the back of each loudmouth asshole's lone neuron he had working as a brain, he heard the whisper, "The cops *have limits* they can't cross. These people *don't*." It was all about respect. We knew this, as did the cops and community.

I know of only one time this silent code was breached. An all-female crew was transporting a male who had been complaining of a headache to the hospital. Suddenly he became confused in the back of the unit, trying to exit the moving vehicle. The petite EMT in the back tried to restrain him, when the confusion exploded into insane rage. Her partner started to pull the bus over, calling for assistance on the police frequency. With this we all started responding in, even with stable patients aboard.

When in trouble, we got a faster response from a police dispatcher than our own. If my partner's life or mine was on the line, we did not have spare seconds to explain our situation. More than once, a foolish crew in trouble didn't get help from our dispatchers, even if they got through.

The bus came to an emergency halt momentarily hidden in an ominous cloud of dark dust and gravel. Its lights pierced the dry dust and the twilight as the sunset. The back door exploded open. The EMT, her blonde hair in disarray, bleeding from nose and mouth, tried to escape the onslaught of the attack. As she jumped for her freedom, two large hands grabbed her from behind in midair. Both she and her attacker crashed to the gravel road. The portable radio, still in its case, smashed into her back and knocked the wind out of her.

Regaining her breath, she tried desperately to fend off the onslaught of the violent blows to her body and head. Pinned to the ground by his weight, trying to wiggle free, she felt her strength being sapped with every powerful blow. Fighting to remain conscious, no longer able to scream, choking from the blood and dry dust, she tried desperately to cover her face. As the unrelenting physical attack continued, she felt his massive hands tear her shirt and bra, pulling them over her head in one swift move.

All her energy faded and she could no longer breathe, realizing she was suffocating. One hand was holding the shirt over her face, as the other hand tightened around her neck. He sensed victory and applied more pressure for the final kill. Now strangling her with one hand, he continued to beat her motionless body with the other. With all strength gone, she started to lapse into unconsciousness, yet her senses intensified. She was aware of the overpowering smell of her own sweat, blood-soaked shirt, and the man's breath. Her body had been exploding in pain, now with the lapsing of consciousness, came a peace she had never known. The EMT realized and accepted she would die. It didn't matter that it was here on this Brooklyn street. What *did* matter *was* the increasing peace and the all-enveloping darkness. As she sensed herself surrendering, feeling the warmth of urine, the pounding fist became duller and more distant.

Her partner waited to hear a confirmation that PD units were on the way. Once confirmed, she rapidly exited the driver's side, running to the back of the unit. As she turned the corner she froze. There was the man on all fours over a lifeless, bloodied, half-nude body.

She screamed and looked for help. A unit watching across the street with two black female EMTs drove away.

As her partner apparently surrendered to death, the tech let out a primordial scream, and attacked. She started beating and kicking the male. With the first blow of the radio, he was roused from his first victim. Turning toward his attacker, he was struck with a flurry of blows, knocking him off his seemingly lifeless victim. His rage was now directed at the partner, who refused to stop the attack. Under an unrelenting onslaught, he now attacked the tech.

The patient ripped the radio from her sweat-soaked hand, smashing her stomach, causing the tech to collapse to her knees. While she was doubled over, unable to catch her breath, he brought the radio up in one final act of savagery and was about to bring it crashing down on the EMT's head.

With the radio in extended hands, the man suddenly lurched forward and the radio continued upward as he let it go, grabbing his back. She heard his heart-stopping scream, as he collapsed to his chest under an onslaught of forceful blows from police officers' nightsticks.

The tech had been knocked to the side by a cop, then dragged to safety as an expanding cloud of pepper mace gas burned everyone's eyes and skin. The male assumed the fetal position under the assault of nightsticks and gas. EMS units arrived as the fray continued, the techs jumping from their moving vehicles. The once quiet street was a turbulent sea of dust, pepper mace gas, and red and white flashing lights. The scream of distant sirens heralded the response of more units.

Guns drawn, the cops cursed and kicked the perpetrator, looking for a response. When none came, they rolled him over on his stomach and handcuffed him. One EMT grabbed the screaming EMT, as she attempted to get to her partner. He held her as she flailed and kicked, cursed, finally collapsing in tears in his arms. A medic knelt beside the unconscious EMT, pulling down the torn, blood-soaked shirt to cover her breasts. He felt for a pulse. At that moment, it seemed like all eternity stood still.

The medic looked into my eyes. With a weary smile he said, "She has a pulse." Everyone said a not-so-silent prayer for her.

The perp went into cardiac arrest on the way into the hospital and the transporting crew worked on him. The escorting police officer did not understand why, after this guy almost killed one of their own, they would try to save his life. The autopsy clearly established that he had a history of headaches. His last headache was from a massive bleed, which resulted in his bizarre behavior. The EMT did recover.

Weapons proliferated at lightning speed. Knives were less common than you might think. Machetes were in vogue. We had numerous jobs where someone had lost an arm or had his intestines hanging out after being sliced by a machete.

On one particular job, we pulled up at the same time as the medics and we walked into the project. At the apartment, a woman in her forties opened the door, smoking her cigarette.

"Hi, did you call?"

Nodding toward the living room without batting an eyelash, "He's in there," she said, walking to the kitchen table and picking up a beer.

Entering the sparsely furnished living room, we saw a black male sitting in a chair, holding a washcloth over his throat.

"Hey, how can we help you?"

He lowered the cloth exposing a cleanly cut trachea.

"Oh, shit. That's cool," one crew member said, while reaching for his intubation kit. The medics argued over who was going to place the tube. The faster hand won. He immediately placed an intubation tube down the cut trachea, inflated the balloon at the end to protect his airway, and used two multi-trauma bandages to stabilize it. Transport to the hospital was uneventful.

EMS Command got wind that crews were now carrying weapons for self-protection. On the streets, law and order was breaking down, and no one was safe. Buses had been shot at, returning to the base with holes in them. Some crews were robbed inside elevators by perps with handguns, though firepower was increasing on the streets to the point of outgunning the cops. My philosophy was if the bastard pulled a gun on us in the elevator there would only be my partner and me alive to fill out the paperwork. It was that fuckin' simple. After Vietnam, and the death of my wife Melanie before our second year together, I wasn't in the mood for some drug-dealing asshole. Thus, I became one with the ghetto mentality and I stayed alive.

One day, one of our African-American chiefs called all King's County units back to the garage. When all the units reported in, he had the following lecture.

"Ladies and gentlemen, I cannot search your cars and definitely not your clothing. Please, do not carry your weapons with you in the ambulance."

Everybody chuckled. Once again an EMS chief had shown his concern for us, right?

Everyone responded, "Chief, we would never do such a thing."

"There's one other issue I want to clear up with you medics," he said in a stern, loud voice. "I don't appreciate no motherfuckin' white paramedic telling my uncle he has African Lipitus!"

Every EMT and paramedic broke up. He walked toward his car, opened the car door, glaring at the paramedics, pointing his finger, and yelled, "Remember what I said, mother fuckers!" He slammed the door and pulled out of the garage.

The event leading up to this little talk involved the medics getting a "Sick" call. As with a majority of the calls, this call was pure bullshit. The patient complained about a cold sore on his lip and felt he deserved special treatment because he was a chief's uncle. Of course, he got special treatment!

Pockets of Hassidic, a sect of Judaism, resided in our area. For the most part, they kept to themselves and preferred the Jewish volunteer ambulance group Hatzolah over EMS.

I'd worked with Hatzolah crews in Brooklyn as well as Manhattan and have certainly seen both ends of the spectrum. I must say that the units up by Columbia Presbyterian Medical Center and in lower Manhattan have proved to be the best.

There were some problems leading to loss of life. In Brooklyn, a black child was left dying, while they worked on a Jewish driver with minor injuries. Also, they tubed a fireman incorrectly, resulting in his death, but nothing of substance happened. If we, on the other hand, refused to help someone, all hell would break loose and we'd be fired, rightfully so.

One night, my unit was on patrol in King's County area when a call came in for an MVA, involving a bus and car. We responded. The people were lucky to get even one bus, given the temperature, call volume, and "EMS crews sabotaging ambulances so they wouldn't have to work."

As we arrived at the designated site, we found a large car in a fender bender with a larger bus. We did a fast survey. The car's passenger and driver, two Hassidics, were not hurt, according to statements made by the driver, who was now rubbing his leg. Almost simultaneously the passenger started rubbing his arm. These "injuries" started when my partner remarked, "Gee, it looks like the guy in the car cut off the bus."

The bus driver was upset because the Eldorado had crossed into his lane in an attempt to make a turn in front of the bus—in essence, cutting it off. Although doing a remarkable job in slowing the bus, so that the impact was minimal, he still had people hurt and paperwork to do. As we observed, some of the passengers started complaining of leg, shoulder, and arm pain and wanted to go to a hospital. Thus we split, I handing out ACRs to the people claiming injuries, my partner taking vital signs.

To call for backup was pointless, since there would be none available. Besides, if the passengers saw more units arriving, it would result in mass hysteria. Their injuries would escalate from being just bounced around, to being unconscious. We had the situation under control though it would have been nice to have someone else to help with the vital signs. More people requested ACRs as they saw the other riders reaching for the forms.

We knew the game as AllStateitis. Claim an injury, go to the hospital, create a paper trail and, sooner or later, you will get a check from the insurance company, especially when the other guy was wrong. In the projects, the people had it down to a science, especially with elevators and falling ceilings.

As we attempted to care for more than twenty people on a bus on a humid night in Brooklyn, tensions rose when the people on the bus realized the people in the car were Hasidim.

"Ladies and gentlemen," I said over the bus PA system, "as you know, EMS is here to serve you. But we need your help."

"Why aren't there more ambulances?"

"Sir, my partner and I sure as hell wish there were more, but that's the mayor's decision. We need your help to ensure everyone gets the paperwork done correctly so we can move you to the hospital."

Everyone listened. "You, young bloods, I want you guys to help the older folks to fill out the paperwork, as my partner takes your vital signs. When he gives you the numbers, write them on the back of the ACR anywhere."

Suddenly, a Hatzolah unit arrived. Exiting the city bus, I greeted the Hatzolah crew, "Listen, could one of you guys help my partner and me for a moment and then we'll help you?" By now the two Hassidics in the car were moaning, putting on a good show.

One Hatzolah tech looked at the all-black occupants of the bus and said, "We don't work on them."

"Okay," I said. I walked back to the bus, noting how the moans had subsided. Back on the bus I grabbed the PA system. "Ladies and gentlemen, I have an announcement. We in EMS are here to serve you. We are understaffed, thanks to an idiot for a mayor and inept leadership in EMS. But we have a problem. I just asked the ambulance that pulled up if one of their crew would be so kind as to help my partner and me. Then we would help them. They wear the same yellow patch as we wear. Yet they said, 'We don't work on them.'"

Several of the younger guys jumped up. There was a lot of cursing.

"Let me finish, please," I said, looking into the eye of one of the young black men, who appeared to be a born leader. He was thin, good looking, very muscular, and wore cutoff jeans, orange work boots, white T-shirt, and a red handkerchief as a dew rag on his head. Gold chains hung from his neck. As I continued to keep eye contact, the man quieted the people. Without taking my eyes off the young man, I continued.

"If you gentlemen would like to step off the bus and have a few words with these folks, fine. Once you are done, you can get back on and finish your paperwork." The young man and several others left the bus and then there were a lot of screams coming from outside.

"What the hell did you do?" asked my partner.

"Listen, no one, but no one wears an EMT patch and then decides who he will help. Let's finish this paperwork then, I'll break it up. Hey, trust me," I said with a smile. My partner laughed and went back to taking vital signs.

A few minutes passed then I called, "Central Three Three Charlie."

"Yes, Three Three Charlie."

"Need a sector, police car, over here, since the people are getting a little upset."

"Are you guys okay?" asked a unit monitoring.

"Oh yeah, we're great, thanks. Safe tour."

"Central, you got the sector coming?"

"Affirmative, one is en route now. I'll put a rush on him."

"Thanks, out." I hopped off the bus and notified the gentlemen, who had three people on the ground and beating the crap out of them, that the cops were inbound. The other guy from the car had run across the street, calling more Hatzolah units and 911.

"Central to Threet Three Charlie."

"Yes, Three Three Charlie here," I answered, as the young warriors filed past my partner and got into their seats.

"We are receiving a call on your job of a riot. Are you guys okay?" It was Mickie, EMS's best dispatcher ever.

"That's a four, I responded with a chuckle." Listening to my voice, she sensed "something" was up.

"I'm sure you are busy, so give me a land line (call on a non-taped phone) after the job," she replied with a chuckle.

"Wilco, out."

My partner was standing next to the bus driver when the two screaming Hatzolah techs followed two police officers, one white, the other Hispanic, onto the bus.

"That's one! There's the others," the mangy, black-bearded, anemic-looking techs screamed, pointing to the young man seated. The cops stepped forward, I blocked the way.

"Hi guys, what's up?"

"Were taking these guys off the bus and charging them and anyone else these guys point out with assault," said the white cop.

"Why? These guys have been here with us, helping fill out paperwork for the older people."

"The whole time?"

"Trust me, yeah," I responded with a smile.

"Look," screamed the Hatzolah tech, trying to push his way past me as I nailed him with an elbow shot in the chest, stopping him in his tracks.

"Look at his wounds! Look at his hands," screamed his partner, as he tried to catch his breath.

"Yeah, look at those hands. If you would have stepped on the bus and did your duty by helping us, you would have seen these wounds," I yelled, grabbing the young black man's bruised and swollen hand, holding it up. "But no. You told me that you and your partner *don't work on them*, whoever the fuck 'them' is."

These were not Manhattan "*Embassy*" cops from the lily-white yuppie "May I open the door for you?" 19th Precinct nor the Central Park "*Squirrel Patrol*" Precinct, but ghetto cops from the 71st Precinct who, like the cops in the 67th, knew the deal. The Hispanic cop wiped the running sweat from his brow, then asked with a knowing smile, "So these guys have been here, correct?"

"Right on. Trust me."

The white cop grabbed the Hatzolah tech and none too gently *helped* him and his friend exit the bus.

"Your precinct captain will hear about this!" one tech screamed at the cop.

"Shut the fuck up or I'll lock your ass up for being stupid!"

"Okay, folks, let's finish this paperwork. This white boy needs some coffee." Everyone laughed.

The young, black male stood up, put out his swollen hand, "You're a cool nigger."

We shook hands, realizing each had reached a new understanding of the other because of the EMS uniform. Life in the ghetto was harsh, at times barbaric, and emotions raw. But it was this very environment of raw, honest emotions that a bigoted person would entrust his child, mother, or wife, to you without question. Neither the police department nor, especially, the fire department had the solemn trust we had. The ghetto cops knew this. On more than one occasion in my career, I've had a cop encourage a junkie, "Tell these guys what you took. They're here to help. We won't arrest you." This trust was earned on the streets by the work of earlier EMTs and paramedics.

Much has been spoken and written about the fire department battling fires in the South Bronx. But Brooklyn was the scene of some horrific fires. Houses, not so much as tenements, turned into instant infernos, trapping people in a heartbeat. Not enough credit had been given to the firefighters who battled these fires. Slum lords charged Haitian illegals several hundred dollars a month to sleep on filthy mattresses in the cellars of these rundown tinderboxes. Each house had in excess of twenty people living in the basement. Talk about Tuberculosis City!

If the house caught fire, these poor souls would be trapped inside. The only hope was the firemen, who aggressively fought these fires, racing against an uncompromising enemy.

One such fire took place on a humid July night. The sun had long disappeared beyond the horizon, but it did nothing to relieve the oppressive heat. Since the front of the bus had no air conditioning, we hung out the windows, to catch a breeze, any breeze. Sweat rolled down our faces. The back of the seats actually made a gushing sound, as our sweat-soaked shirts glided against a layer of dampness. My green pants were soaked in the butt and crotch as I tried in vain to find some relief for my cramped legs. Then we received the call for a standby at a fire.

With lights on, the sirens pierced into the night, deafening and hurting both our ears. Another year passed before EMS would be called on the carpet by OSHA (Office of Safety and Health Administration) and ordered to remove the sirens from the tops of the vehicles and place them into the forward grillwork. Even after this mandate, we had to be insubordinate. Officers, without enough ambulances, ordered us to take them into service. More than once I was threatened, but nothing ever came of it.

As we raced along, a car cut in front of us. Each time I attempted to maneuver, this idiot cut us off like it was a big fuckin' game. Finally I got the upper hand and almost put him into two parked cars. I slowed him down, as we broke off of Utica Avenue and headed toward Brownsville. As we flew up dilapidated Livonia Avenue, the sound of the passing overhead train was drowned out by our wailing siren. The landscape was one of despair, magnified a thousandfold by the stripped cars and burned-out shells of buildings. Children as young as six, almost naked, wandered aimlessly on the torn concrete streets.

We continued past rat-infested lots strewn with garbage. Previously, we had been called to remove bodies from these lots. The half-flesh-covered remains still had their hands tied behind them. Could these be called human remains after flies, maggots, dogs, and rats feasted on them?

Two women, one of them very pregnant, shared a large bottle of beer, cigarettes glowing wistfully in the night. Behind them, two children, one about six and the other younger, played with a bottle they took off an unconscious shit- and urine-covered drunk on the sidewalk.

"Hey, here comes this asshole again," Joe yelled. Sure enough, the lunatic driver was at it again, but this time I was ready as Joe braced for what he knew what was coming. At the count of three, the brakes locked up. The pursuing driver locked his brakes, causing him to swerve sideways, momentarily losing control and sending his car into a railway support beam. The passenger door was totally destroyed, as we accelerated, wiping the sweat from our eyes.

At the scene, we found two houses were infernos. It was complete chaos. The red, orange, and yellow flames formed gigantic tongues thirty feet tall, lapping at a star-filled sky. Dancing orange cinders from the burning buildings created a surreal light show as they fell.

Against this backdrop of hell, firemen screamed at people not to jump, as they attempted to rescue them with ladders. A fireman started up one ladder to get to a woman on the roof, who was holding a small bundle. He hadn't gotten up more than five feet, when the wall collapsed. The ladder disappeared along with the fireman in a black cloud of smoke illuminated by burning cinders. Suddenly there was a gigantic belch of orange flame, leaping into the sky, followed by more collapse.

The woman on the roof, barefoot in a sheer nightgown, disappeared into a ball of flame. Her last desperate act was to throw the bundle free. A cop ran for the bundle, as other firemen hosed down their brother pulled from the collapse.

Other units responded and the MERV (Major Emergency Response Vehicle) pulled up. In those days, the county MERV was nothing more than a large bread truck converted to hold extra stretchers, oxygen bottles, and the like. Other MERVs were modified schoolbuses. All were manned by one driver, an EMT, and once on the scene would usually be manned by two paramedics from a responding unit, along with two EMTs.

In the chaos, as we got our equipment together, the car that had kept cutting us off pulled up. The driver locked eyes with my partner, evidently recognizing the bus number. Jumping out of the car, running, arms flailing and cursing at us, he was met in mid-sentence with a fist that knocked him to the ground. Both of us had dropped our equipment, ready to take turns adjusting this guy's attitude and covering each other's backs. The man got up slow and grabbed a piece of wood, drawing it up. A man from the crowd screamed his name. He turned and the stranger started yelling at him in his native Haitian language. It was only then he dropped the stick, raised his hands and fell to his knees, screaming. His friend dragged the half-conscious, bleeding man away.

Joe asked, "What's this asshole's problem?"

"He's not an asshole because he is black," the man responded with indignation. "He is upset because he and his family lived in that house," the man said as he pointed to the blazing inferno. "Perhaps you should stop insulting him because he is black and do your job," he retorted with disdain.

Joe stepped toward the man but I put my hand up and with the other grabbed the Haitian's shoulder spinning him around to face me.

"Listen, Stymie, before you talk to my partner about us doing our job, perhaps you should ask your Dick Head friend what took us so long?" The Haitian tried to break free, but I increased my grip till the man stopped moving, now grimacing in pain. The Haitian glared, the leaping flames of hatred reflected in his eyes. His brown skin glistened with sweat, as he flinched each time a cinder landed on him.

"Now that I have your full fuckin' attention, ask that piece of worthless shit why he cut us off at Utica Avenue? Ask him who's laughing now, shithead?"

Joe and I picked up our gear without another word and responded to the EMS patrol boss.

A fireman yelled they were bringing out six people, including four children. A medic yelled for the patients to be brought to him, as he directed the police to push back the crowd.

The firemen carried out body after body. For the children, the individual fireman did mouth-to-mouth as they approached the medic's location. The male medic called for all the intubation tubes and more BVMs.

I got an idea and, against the burning, crackling inferno, grabbed the body off the fireman, placing the person on the littered street corner, positioning the heads of the adults to hang over the sidewalk corner, to give the medic better visual access for placing the breathing tubes. Both medics, male and female, were on their stomachs on the dirty gutter, intubating patients.

Alongside a medic, Joe bent over the body, doing compressions then several ventilations on the adult, before moving to the next adult. The female directed me and a cop to stay with the four kids, ranging from two months to twelve years, and keep bagging and ventilating them till help arrived. The white cop talked to the children we were working desperately to save. Tears ran down his sweat- and soot-covered face, cascading into a gutter now awash with water from the fire hydrant.

People with various injuries and burns were lined up as units pulled in. The smell of burned flesh hung in the air, permeating your very skin. Two at a time, children were loaded onto long boards and then strapped into place, in an attempt not to displace the intubation tubes. The arriving EMTs listened and worked with the two medics, leaving the scene in separate buses with the children as fresh medics took over the care of the other intubated adults. These were quickly evacuated out of the area. We then were directed to open our bus and prepare to treat patients, since the MERV was inundated.

A woman held the hand of her eight-year-old son, who was carrying his two-year-old sister. The woman spoke little English, but you didn't need an interpreter to see she was burned. Her cheap, silk nightgown was melted to her legs and chest. Joe worked quickly to check her airway and strip her of non-attached clothing, cooling surface skin areas with sterile water. We observed first- and second-degree burns on her upper thighs, abdomen, and back of the neck. Pink flesh showed where the fire had burned her brown skin. The children were fine. A patrol boss decided to move her to another unit that was heading to a burn center.

As things were winding down, cops carried a forty-year-old male who broke his leg and suffered minor burns as he ran with a police officer to save the bundle. The bundle was a six-month-old baby girl who had suffered smoke inhalation and a skull fracture. Both the little girl and the police officer who had also suffered smoke inhalation and burns to his hands were removed to King's County.

The man was loaded into the back of our unit and I started to check him over. His ten-year-old son also came on board, telling me his mom worked at the hospital. Once I was satisfied that the man was stable, comfortable and on oxygen, I strapped the boy into the seat.

The man had asked that his wife be notified so she could pick up their son. "No problem, sir." I saw the concern on the son's face as his dad closed his eyes, breathing in the oxygen. Wiping the sweat from the patient's brow, I looked at the boy. "You should be very proud. Your dad is a real hero. He'll be fine." This got a smile.

At King's County, I called the boy's mother. She was on her way. The once noisy, congested corridors of this city hospital were empty. The little boy sat alone in the harsh, sterile light, while doctors in the crash room examined his father. I got two cans of Pepsi Cola and walked back into the quiet waiting room. The silence was broken only by the moan of the father, as the doctors worked and the janitor emptied the garbage cans.

Sitting next to the little boy, I opened the sodas and handed him one.

We both took a sip but then the little boy looked into my eyes. His brown skin was covered in sweat, a blue-and-yellow, striped shirt was ripped and covered in soot. I reached over without saying a word, put my arm around the boy, and pulled him close as the child softly cried. There we sat in silence. When the mother arrived a few moments later, the little boy jumped up and ran to her saying, "Don't worry, Mom, Dad's a hero." The mother thanked me, as I shook the hand of the little boy.

Outside the hospital, I found my partner with other crews milling around. Two medics sat further down the ramp on the wall. The young blonde had her knees pulled up to her chest, arms around her legs. She was crying. Her partner sat silently next to her, with his arm around her. We walked silently past them, toward the garage. As we approached the garage, Joe headed for his car and I passed the office, noticing the duty officer talking to someone. I recognized the Haitian we had read the riot act to. The lieutenant waved me in.

What the fuck, I thought. Completely drained, covered in sweat, soot and spots of blood, I trudged into the office. "Yeah?"

"Mr. Dubow wishes to tell you something, Schrang."

"I just want to tell you that Leon lost his wife and six-month-old daughter whom you and your partner were racing to save."

With this, he put out his hand. I shook it, turned, and walked out. There were no words to say.

I did rolling stops till I entered the Interborough Parkway, accelerating my red Honda, downshifting to enter Dead Man's Curve. Coming out, I looked at Rene's plot of fresh dirt on the hill. Rene was a young patient, a friend who died. Once leaving Cypress Hills Cemetery, coming out of a slight turn, I accelerated. The cool freshness from the Forest Park trees enveloped me like a cleaning dip in the ocean.

Rising in front was Great Grandmother Moon in all her glory. The deeper I drove into the woods heading toward Queens, the more the sweet fragrance of the flowers soaked every pore. Tears rolled down my filthy face.

Christmas was the season to be jolly. We brought gifts and piled them into the drum we'd set up at King's County. I kept a list of the kids we took care of during the year and loaded the bus, making special stops for little people during the tour. The dispatcher, Mickie, worked around us while we made our merry rounds.

Lieutenant Friszell called Barry and me into the office after we made our run. "Listen, go get some eggnog for the crews."

"Yeah, like we are going to find eggnog in East New York at this hour?"

"Get your ass out there and don't come back without the eggnog." Oh the love that flowed from this man. Then he added, "*Remember,* this is the birthday of Baby Jesus. So please, no trouble tonight." Trouble us? Barry and me? Oh perish the thought.

East New York during the early eighties was not a place where too many people cared about the birth of Jesus or Santa. Hell, as far as most were concerned, a white man riding into the neighborhood was fair game with or without reindeer. If East New York was depressing during the day, it digressed into a venomous, parasitical world where the strong feasted on the weak. Just as the foam of beer is hidden within the body as it is poured, so to these shadows of society's darkest side hid many amongst the hardworking people during the daylight hours. But just like the foam, they rose after the people locked their doors. Now in this ghost land of crushed souls, the invisible became the only visible reality. Cops and EMS both were no less part of the ghetto than the dealer, or the eleven-year-old cracker (crack addict) selling herself. And just like them, we, both services, paid a price.

We finally found a grocery store about to close. I stood at the counter near a freezer with dingy glass doors about waist high. To my left was the window to the store and behind me were some dilapidated shelves. An elderly, black woman brought up some items and whispered to me, "Look out for a setup." She was referring to four black young warriors of the street who had entered several minutes prior.

"Now Merry Christmas to you too, young lady," I said, looking toward Barry near the cold drink section. Two of the young warriors came up to me.

"Yo, got some change?" I had already figured the one closest was going to kiss Mister Softy when I put his head through the case. The second asshole was going through the window to my left. Barry already knew his prey. The hunters were about to become the hunted.

In the most Christian season of humility, I responded, "Fuck off." Folks, this is East New York, not cupcake East Side Manhattan, or Long Island. On these streets the perps were better armed than the cops. Here, a look would lead to death from an acute case of lead poisoning (gunshot) and no one would care as they rifled your body for change. Thus, EMS crews needed to control the situation through the gift of talking and, when all else failed, letting them know they may win in killing you, but they *can't afford the cost.* They might have the weapon, but I accepted death long ago on a hillside in Vietnam. They were still afraid of death, I wasn't. Thus I had what the cops call "officer presence."

"Yo, mother! You want some of us?" the poor fool asked.

"Okay, asshole. Not here, outside." That was our Christmas gift to this hardworking, black owner who was trying to make a living. Once outside, the four chumps lined up with their backs against the beautiful glass.

"Think you tough?" asked one asshole, his head tilting to the side.

"Yep," I said, stepping on his toe, turning my baseball hat sideways, slowly tilting my head to the side so as to look him in the eyes. "We're going to kick your motherfuckin' ass, then take you and the girls here to the hospital before you go to central booking, so swing," I added, making the point of inserting my trigger finger into his chest.

All of a sudden I heard Barry say, "*Remember* Baby Jesus. *Remember* Baby Jesus and his birthday," a reference to Lieutenant Friszell. I was trying not to smile since I had my war face on.

This little band of warriors started talking sense to the fool. In the end, the County had its eggnog and Baby Jesus had another birthday. The bodega was intact. The little warriors would live another night to rob, rape, and pillage. As for us, we had gotten respect, laughing as we drank the special eggnog, and Barry kept repeating, "Remember Baby Jesus."

TWO

EMS What a Mess

The Civilian Gods (EMS Chiefs)

As EMTs and paramedics served the public on the streets of New York, making do with the least, the chiefs had interesting times. Rumors mounted with scandal after scandal. If it wasn't the outside vendor which was "fixing" broken windows on ambulances it was about an Assistant District Attorney's car reportedly broken into as it sat in clear view outside EMS Headquarters in Maspeth, Queens. Files needed for an EMS corruption investigation were reportedly taken during the break-in.

We remembered a certain "individual" going from garage to garage in a panic mode checking to ensure that the *books,* our time sheets, were correct. A smiling lieutenant said, "It was to ensure we were not carrying anyone on the payroll who was no longer there, but still getting paid."

The rumors flew about theft of services, being paid when not present, kickbacks from vendors.

Certain chiefs, like Joel Friedman, tried to do what was right for his people and the public. At times he would have crews set up tables to take blood pressures. It wasn't much, but it gave him a reputation of caring for the community. He was the rarity, but in the end, he too folded under the pressure of egotistical, inept managers referred to as "the gods."

The EMS God, in this case, Robert Becker, relied on a special unit called ISU (Inspectional Services Unit) to keep the pressure on field personnel. This, coupled with the CCU (Civilian Complaint Unit), allowed certain people to go on witch-hunts and personal vendettas. The EMS crews believed neither group was there to help, but rather both were there to screw us.

One medic spoke to me of his unit having been "tailed" by an ISU all day. The wannabe detectives drove an unmarked civilian car. The crew received a call for a "'Difficult Breather" at the local precinct. After evaluating the patient, they spewed out their frustrations to two officers. One of them, the precinct captain, listened intently as the crew waited for an escort to the hospital with a sick prisoner. The captain had great sympathy for EMS crews, since he knew they were abused by the public, but more so by their own supervision.

He remembered in his earlier years he had lain on the roof of a tenement, shot in his stomach. He had volunteered for the elite Narcotics Undercover Unit on a routine "buy and bust" narcotic street operation. Something went wrong and he was shot. He recalled the feeling of being alone as the firefight swirled around him. Dying on the roof, he was saved by an unknown medic and EMT who rushed through the hail of gunfire to work on him. He spent several months in and out of the hospitals, never learning their names. But he never forgot about them.

After bringing their patient/prisoner to the hospital, the medics received a "Cardiac Condition" and responded deep in Harlem. As they pulled up to the job, the crew spotted the unmarked car at the curb at the end of the block. Both paramedics had had enough. After evaluating the patient, one medic asked if he could use the family's phone. The wife showed the medic the phone in the kitchen and returned to her husband.

"911, what is your emergency?"

"I was just threatened with a gun and robbed," said the medic into the phone, adding a black man's accent to his voice.

"Where? Can you describe them? Are they still there?"

"Yo think I'm some dumb-ass nigger? Sure I can. They're still sitting in the car and gots a big-ass gun. They says they cops and flashed the tin at me before takin' my money."

The medic gave the description of the car, the two "perps" and their location, and repeated the size of the gun. Hanging up the phone, he returned to help his partner who was now packaging the patient in the stair chair.

As they carried the patient out the front door, they heard the wailing sirens of the approaching police cars. They carried the patient down the turn-of-the-century steps. On the sidewalk, both looked up the block, as the sectors, along with unmarked crime units, came to a screeching halt all around the unsuspecting ISU vehicle. The medics had loaded the patient and the wife into the back of the bus. Up the block the two wannabe "detectives" were face down and spread-eagle on the hood of their car. A police captain stepped forward from the sea of gun-drawn cops and said something to his officers. The duo were cuffed and unceremoniously forced from the hood of their car onto the ground.

"Them cops are doing a good job," said the old lady.

"Yeah, they sure are," said the medic with a big smile, as he looked at his partner who had made the call.

"What?" said the medic, who was also smiling as he closed the door. Walking up to the front of the bus, he savored his deed. The police captain stepped over the ISU crew and smiled as he watched the bus pull away. There is indeed street justice. Sometimes, just sometimes, it needs a little help.

Meanwhile on the streets in another part of EMS land, Barry Travis and I got called to a "Jumper Up." On arrival, we saw a black female standing on a small ledge of a twelve-story building. I asked Barry if he wanted to go up, but he said he would wait for her to come down, one way or the other, thank you. I took my tech bag and started upstairs.

On the roof, two black males talked to the troubled woman. She was standing on an outer, six-inch ledge. To get to this precarious perch she had climbed over a four-foot wall on the roof, so only mid-chest up was visible. Two cops from the Sixty-seventh Precinct remained about four feet away, pleading with her to come in and talk.

Approaching, one officer and I made eye contact. Looking over the side of the red brick building, I thought she picked a cool spot; the view of Brooklyn was really great, and there was a breeze. Directly below her, stood a lone, beautiful tree, cars, my unit. Barry was rapping to some girls, as an EMS patrol boss pulled up. Slowly the crowd of several hundred became an ugly wave of insanity. They were screaming in unison, "Jump, bitch! Jump!" As the wave of humanity lunged to and fro, a carnival atmosphere took over as the sporadic chant became a thunderous roar, for the woman to kill herself.

Standing there surveying the insanity, an ESU (Emergency Service Unit) of the police department came to the roof with equipment. These guys are the specialists who gain entry into an apartment, remove trapped motorists, or when under fire, have the extra firepower to ruin a perp's day.

As they put on their harnesses, I looked over at this pudgy ghetto cop from the Sixty-seventh Precinct. I turned my attention to the woman and then back to him. We both *knew* in that split second she would not wait for ESU to bring her in. As the crowd came to a fevered pitch, screaming, "Jump, bitch. Jump," she turned on the ledge so she could jump out past a tree, which would have broken her fall. She was dead serious wanting a confirmed kill by landing on the cars and, hopefully, not my unit below. This girl was serious, but so were we. As if we had been one person, the cop lunged, shoving past the two men talking and gripped her arms as she turned, screaming, "I want to die!"

At the same moment, I shoved one of the men out of my way, jumped up, and straddled the wall. The crowd roared as I bent over the side of the building, grabbing between her legs with one hand, holding on to the roof with my other. The cop held on for dear life and pulled. He was short in physical stature, but not in courage. He prevented her from pulling him over the ledge with her as I managed, by the grace of God, to flip her back onto the roof. ESU came running; still, she fought as they cuffed her. The two idiot friends shrieked, "You're hurting her!"

Once she was cuffed, one ESU cop looked at me, eyes glaring, "Couldn't wait, could you?"

I looked at the cop who was brushing off his uniform. He heard the exchange and walked over.

"Hey man, don't waste your time thinking about those assholes. Thanks for helping me. I really thought I was going to lose her."

I looked over the ledge at the dispersing crowd and wondered who was really insane?

Downstairs, we loaded her into the back of the ambulance. The patrol boss came up to me wearing his white helmet. Our helmets were orange and stored in plastic in the vehicle. After witnessing everything from below, he said, "I should do paperwork on you for that stunt."

I honestly thought he was talking about an award or something, but then he continued. "That is not part of your job title. Do you realize I could write you up for endangering yourself and not having your helmet on?"

Now I understood.

He was more concerned about doing paperwork than on saving a person's life. He was no better than the crowd who screamed for her blood.

"Fuck you and your helmet, asshole."

"What did you say?"

"Hey, Barry, let's get out of here, before I stuff him in his fuckin' helmet."

I got in the unit with the jumper and the cop slammed the door behind me. Needless to say, no paperwork was ever generated, but I learned. EMS chiefs were in the business to ensure no one knew how dangerous our job was. They would go to any extreme to keep the press from finding out. If it hit the press, there would be substance to the union's claim we had a dangerous job, thus costing the city more in pay and wages. Hell, as far as the EMS chiefs were concerned, we were just ambulance drivers and civilians directed by the EMS god.

Aside from the usual blood-and-guts runs, we also got medical jobs. Sixteen-year-old Rene, who was dying of leukemia, stuck in my heart.

The first time I went to his home to pick him up, I liked him. He was wasting away and the pain was unbearable. He lived with his mother, grandmother, and three sisters. He loved reggae music and promised to take me to a concert when he got better. But Rene did not get better. The pain increased day by day, hour by hour. Week after week, we were called.

If another unit was called, I'd get the okay from my partner and take the call from the other unit. It got so bad Rene made his final trip to King's County. Before and after work, I went to the floor where he was spending his final hours. The room was barren except for his bed. The window was open without a screen, allowing the flies to enter. The paint was peeling off the walls. Rene lay in all sorts of contorted positions, his face emaciated, crying, and moaning unintelligible words. Sometimes I would sit and talk to him. In the end, I could only stand in the doorway and whisper a prayer through my tears. God, how much I hurt for him, for his family. After what seemed an eternity, he died. I attended his funeral on a rainy day and drove the kids home.

Driving near Dead Man's Curve, on the hill, you could see, by a lone tree, Rene's burial plot in Cypress Hills Cemetery. I really missed that kid.

We were frequently called to a young black girl named Resheida. She was a thirteen-year-old beauty with sickle cell disease, in which the red blood cells, instead of being round, are shaped like a sickle or half-moon. They clump and form blockages, causing extreme pain. This child waited for me because I'd pamper her by carrying her to the unit.

She was so intelligent and had a knowing smile. Her mother was blessed to have a child of such courage. All who met Resheida were instantly disarmed by her smile. I can't ever remember her crying or being down about the disease.

That's the nature of the beast in this job. We met people at their worst moments, spent twenty or thirty minutes with them, and then we were gone, leaving nothing but a memory.

Barry and I were assigned a "Sick" job. We pulled up to the specified destination and checked all four corners. It was a beautiful summer day with people milling about, but no one approached the ambulance. Finally, I got on the PA, "Did anyone call for an ambulance?"

"Your mother," came a response from a group of teens sitting on a wall.

"Is anyone hurt or sick, and needing an ambulance?"

"Yo, mother fucker. Your mother a ho (whore) and sucks dick," came the response, as they sat laughing, drinking beer.

I had almost enough, "You're right about my mother. But at least I know who my father is."

Barry dove for the floor, as the teens ran toward the unit, throwing bottles. He screamed, "Are you fuckin' crazy? They'll kill us!"

As I accelerated the bus around the block, Barry finally rose from the floorboard and sat upright in the seat, until I made another turn.

"Where are you going? Oh noooo, you . . ."

He didn't have time to finish his statement as the ambulance pulled up parallel to the crowd of teens. In a split second, I turned the gas-powered ignition on and off, back firing the ambulance! Teens dove to the ground, screaming they were being shot! As we left the area, I contacted the dispatcher, telling her there was no patient, but we did have respect, and for me, well, I had satisfaction.

With the increased call volume, EMS was expanding and getting new ambulances. The gods wanted more lieutenants, but for whatever reason, they decided to have acting lieutenants. These folks were promised the world, but took it in the end from the chiefs.

In 1984–85, we had the actors. One noted actor was an EMT, whom we named Loradicka. Once the bars were on, he thought he was General Patton sitting at the desk wearing a starched uniform decorated with medals up the wazoo.

Concerning medals in EMS, you had to write yourself up. Chief Becker got the Medal of Honor for remaining at Location One, Headquarters, Puzzle Palace, during a bomb threat. They cleared the place of a damn paint can. Another version of the story told of a minor fire in the building and he reportedly went in to get out his brother. Whichever one it was, he had to write himself up for this nonsense.

One idiot medic from Bellevue jumped in the East River after her partner jumped in to save a patient. The problem was, the idiot could not swim. When asked why she did it, she said, "It seemed like the right thing to do." Unfortunately, her partner had to save the patient and her. This inept individual, who wasn't much of a medic anyway, reportedly got a medal and wound up going on to work with the CCU.

Getting back to our other hapless hero, Loradicka, seated at attention, answered the phone, "Station Three Three Acting Lieutenant Loradicka, sir!" Chief Becker called to check up on his little acting lieutenant.

Everyone was tired of this idiot. One day, I removed the mouthpieces from the phones in the office and walked outside to make a call, pretending to be the chief. But before I could call, the chief actually called. Here was poor Loradicka pleading into the dead phone that he could hear but couldn't talk. With his chances fading of becoming one of "Becker's Peckers," he attempted to think.

But never let it be said he wasn't resourceful. "Take out the mouthpieces, will you?" He found the solution by having his own personal headset plugged into the phone. Sitting behind his desk, he looked like a Burger King worker with a chest full of French, not Liberty, fries above his spit-shined shield that looked even less dignified than a security guard's.

In those days, we could turn a knob and talk point-to-point on the radio without the dispatcher ever hearing us. We had a lot of fun sitting behind a unit, calling them, and assigning them bogus jobs. But I could do better than that for the actor.

Outside the garage, we all sat as I went point-to-point. Acting Lieutenant Loradicka sat at attention behind his desk, surveying his empire, feeling like a junior god, an almost Becker Pecker. Awaiting a call from the head god, he emulated him by having his radio on, volume up, monitoring all that was happening in his universe. His call sign was 333.

Over the radio he didn't need to say "Acting" 333. Here on the radio, Acting Lieutenant Loradicka was in charge.

As such, he felt a rush when giving orders over the radio, which he often did. All was peaceful and content in his part of the universe until a bloodcurdling scream came over his radio.

"Central! Central! Emergency! Three Thirty-three just had a heart attack. Send help!"

Our hero jumped up screaming into his radio, "Three Thirty-three! I'm okay."

"Unit calling?" the dispatcher asked.

Again, point- to-point, "He's dying. Oh God, send the medics!"

With this, Loradicka jumped up and ran toward the Dutch doors to get better reception in the garage area. Suddenly his neck violently snapped back as the headset was still attached to the phone which flew off, hitting him in the eye. The phone crashed onto the floor with a thud and a ring. Moving fast, holding his right eye and radio, he crashed into the lower half of the Dutch door, which was closed. His first point of contact was with his genitals into the doorknob, the second point of contact was his right leg as he hit the door. Over the top he was catapulted. His third point of contact was his head hitting the garage floor. Out came a bloodcurdling scream. His last point of contact was when the rest of his body caught up with his head. The annoyed dispatcher asked, "Three Thirty-three, do you have a message?"

"Oh, God," he went, whimpering in excruciating pain, "I'm . . . I'm . . . fine."

Ignoring the buffoon, the now agitated dispatcher asked, "Anyone in the area of the County, *please* respond to see what's going on with Three Thirty-three! The tour commander has been calling him on the land line and no one is answering." Well, units did respond to find the hapless acting lieutenant slightly hurt.

One day at roll call, Hawk Eye commanded, "Schrang, follow me. I want to talk to you."

He headed for the men's bathroom.

"That's very sweet," I said with a smile, "but I like girls." Everyone laughed.

"Get your ass in here now!"

Walking behind him, I started to unzip my pants for all to see. Upon entering, Hawk Eye stood facing the urinal, doing his thing as I waited.

"Listen, I know you have been pulling a lot of shit around here, but you have just gone too far."

"What are you talking about?"

"Look, I just got a phone call from the cops that Lieutenant Loradicka—"

"That's 'acting,'" I interrupted.

"Yeah, the idiot was pulled over on Eastern Parkway because some wise ass put hospital police license plates on his car." At this point, Hawk Eye laughed so hard urine ran down his pants. "Shit!" His laughter was contagious.

"I would never do such a thing," I said, laughing, walking out of the men's room, winking at the crews. Hawk Eye finally came out, his pants wet. Everyone looked as I zipped my pants, "Well, that scared the piss out of him." Everyone except Hawk Eye howled.

Acting Lieutenant Loradicka had a habit of literally flying out of the garage in his command car. On more than one occasion, he almost hit crew members walking into the garage. Hawk Eye was on a rampage, screwing anyone for anything to make his brownie points so he could become a captain.

One crew figured they could get rid of both for the price of one. So with the blessing of the crews, they watched, learned, and planned. Loradicka always parked his car in the same place, across from the inside pumps at the county garage. Behind said vehicle ran a wide pipe. One day, a crew tied a rope from the rear axle to the pipe. It was calculated that only Hawk Eye would be in the office when Lieutenant Loradicka took off. It was also calculated how many feet it would take before the rear axle broke off, sending the old command cab hurtling out of control with Loradicka at the wheel, hitting the gas pumps, killing the actor and Hawk Eye in the resulting explosion and fire. The upside, they'd be dead and we would get a new facility. All was set until some MVO (Motor Vehicle Operator) warned them, and they found the rope.

Another actor with a bad attitude came to the county. One night, he pulled up to his home in Staten Island. He was tired after a day of abusing crews and writing them up for nonsense.

He got out of his car and gazed at the ranch-style home. His mother-in-law had been very useful in putting most of her savings into the house so he could afford the mortgage. She was as easy a swindle as the bitch he married. The house looked quiet with the living room light coming from behind the crisp, clean curtains. Taking in a deep breath, he exhaled in satisfaction as he reached to place the key in the door. The front door light was out. Now he would have a reason to smack the bitch around. God help her if she didn't have the food ready, he thought.

"Hey," he attempted to speak as a large, gloved hand covered his mouth. He felt the cold steel of a barrel under his ear and froze in terror.

"People are tired of your fuckin' fat ass messing with us County Mounties," said a voice colder than the barrel. "Look to your right, bastard," the voice whispered. As his eyes turned, he saw the barrel and started to whimper. He shut his eyes as tears rolled down his fat cheeks. Holding them closed in an effort to make all this go away, he shook uncontrollably.

"Cut the shit, bastard, or I'll do you right now," the voice was getting angrier. "Remember, I know where you live. I also know how you enjoy beating your wife. Keep fucking with us and the little woman will be my ho. I'll enjoy her as well as your insurance money."

The actor was becoming dizzy. "Don't move or open your eyes till you can't hear the sound of my car." The intruder knew he would not have to be told twice. The actor did as he was told. He became a model officer until his transfer came through within a week.

One non-acting new lieutenant went to the Liberty Outpost on Pennsylvania Avenue, a fort in a wasteland of humanity. Coming in from

Manhattan with a real piss-and-vinegar attitude, he eyed slots for captain then chief. One day, he found his private car, which was parked inside the garage. The windows were broken, sugar was in the gas tank, and tires were flattened. A sign read, "Now you can leave," one of his favorite sayings as a "boss." Needless to say, he went to another station.

One of the real pleasures of the job was meeting people of exceptional talent. In the early eighties, as a County Mountie, I met one such person, EMT Vinny McMichael. Vinny was a tall, astute, soft-spoken black man. He introduced me to his wonderful sister and to his artistic talent. Lieutenant Friszell was so impressed, he had Vinny paint the New York City skyline with EMS logo on the inside garage door at the station. Vinny designed a vibrant and colorful city scene.

One day while we were working together, Vinny paid me the ultimate compliment. Things were really getting bloody in Brooklyn and he was very concerned about the safety of his sister. As we sat drinking sodas he became somber, "If we pulled up to the scene and my sister was shot, I'd want you to work on her." To this day I am still honored that he thought that much of my ability as an EMT. Vinny was a gifted painter and a true professional, his sister, a ravishing African-American beauty.

One night, we pulled up to a gentleman who was having chest pains. I drove as Vinny took care of the patient. The white patient became adamant that he did not want Vinny to touch him because Vinny was black. When I got the picture I told the guy we were leaving. No one would talk to my partner with such ignorance. I'd let the bastard die in his hatred. Vinny reminded me of our job to help all. He demonstrated his love by stepping back and insisting I aid the bigoted patient. I did and was grateful for the lessons both taught me.

The police officers, for the most part, were hardworking, honest cops. Most did not live in the neighborhood, but felt it was theirs and served their extended family in honor. I liked the sixty-seventh and seventy-first precincts. Long before the Seventy-seventh Precinct became known for its bad cops, we knew about them and others.

One night my partner and I rolled on a "Shooting" in a bodega. We pulled up at the same time as the sector. The doorknob to the bodega turned easily as no lock was in place. We entered the store, crouching low behind the cops, their weapons drawn. A black male in his twenties was behind the Plexiglas, neither seeing nor hearing our entrance.

"Freeze, motherfucker!" screamed an officer, as he stood up in front of the Plexiglas partition. He pointed his weapon through the opening and aimed at the man's chest two feet away. The guy glanced at the black revolver. "Do it, shithead, and I'll blow your motherfuckin' brains out!" His partner and I pushed in the small door with force, as his partner provided cover. Inside, as the officer covered my back, I shoved the male to the waiting officer. While he kissed the floor, we checked two adjacent rooms, which were clear.

Behind the counter, we saw a three-foot-high shelf stacked with clear bags containing white powder. The shelf was covered with bags stacked three rows high. On top was the thirty-eight, its six-inch black barrel in stark contrast to the pure white "snow," Cocaine or cleanser? At the back of the shelf, I saw money stacked, more than I'd ever seen except on TV shows like *Miami Vice*.

The cop and I glanced at each other, as a black sergeant walked in. His uniform was unseemly pressed for this warm Brooklyn night.

"Get the cuffs off him and everybody outside," he curtly ordered, "and close the door."

The two cops looked at him, his glare alone could kill.

Outside, I leaned up against the door, which I had left partially open.

"Give me the name," the sergeant asked the man who was no longer handcuffed. That's how long the sergeant was on the scene. The name was spoken and I pulled back as the sergeant opened the door arrogantly, strutting out. Standing erect, his hat squarely planted on his head, a thin black mustache meticulously trimmed. Realizing I had been listening, he stared. His eyes were empty and black, void of emotion, but I stared back. Without breaking the stare, he commanded, "It's a ninety." This meant unfounded, nothing was there

Both cops started to protest, "Sarge. What do you mean unfound . . ."

He turned his frigid stare on them.

"Get in your vehicles now. It's a ninety," he hissed in a cold, hollow tone. We all got into our vehicles.

"Let's go back to King's County," I said to my partner. As we pulled away, I saw the sergeant standing with his arms crossed, watching me. Back at King's County, I consulted with a friend, BJ.

"Forget what you saw. The whole damn precinct is bought. If you try to take it anywhere, EMS will give out your home address and you'll be set up or killed."

I knew all too well how EMS rolled over, giving up home addresses of their employees. I also knew that a rival dealer had set up the guy in the bodega. That's why the door was open and the call came in about someone shot. It was the worst drug deal I saw in a precinct.

While Vinny went to get some dinner, I sat in the bus, watching a guy on a motorcycle. He flew up and down the block with little regard for safety, almost causing a couple of accidents. I knew what was coming. Sure enough, the overweight Italian ended up on his fat ass in the middle of the street. Slowly covering my coffee, putting on my sunglasses, I got out of the vehicle, and walked over to him. He was flat on his back, looking like a beached Sicilian whale

"Sir, before I ask you if you are hurt," I said in a calm soothing voice, "I have to tell you I have been watching you and sir, you're a real asshole. Now that I've said that, I feel better. If you're hurt, I'll be happy to help you."

He grumbled something about not being hurt, except for his pride, got up and limped alongside his bike down the block. Gee, and then people wonder why I call motorcyclists "organ donors."

A police pursuit of three armed men who had just robbed a store on Utica Avenue was in progress!

"Shots fired," the pursuing sector screamed into the radio. "They're heading toward the Parkway, Eastern Parkway."

Units were running from the Seventy-first Precinct trying to cut off the vehicle, but these guys were fast. We had been monitoring and decided to assist. With lights and sirens on, we went into hyperspeed, until we hit gridlocked traffic. Four blocks ahead, we saw the police car with lights flashing chasing a gray Corvette. Both were weaving in and out of traffic. Some cars were jumping sidewalks to get out of the way of what appeared to be a deranged driver. The ground was littered with packages and broken bottles, dropped by horrified pedestrians fleeing for safety. Other cars came to a screeching halt to rubberneck. It was total chaos and great to be part of!

I grabbed for the PA system, not wanting to miss the action.

"Okay, move it, right, everyone. Let's clear a path." No one moved. The car directly in front of us sat there and the driver viewed the crew in his mirror with a blank look on his face. This outraged both Vinny and me!

"Hey you! Yeah, you! Move the damn vehicle now!" Still nothing happened, but the driver's face appeared even more stupid.

"Hey, you with the dreadlocks! Pull them out of your damn ears, deflate your fuckin' lips so you can see, and move the motherfuckin' car!"

As I attempted to adjust my grip on the PA mike, I suddenly realized nothing was coming from the PA. A closer examination of my hand led to the discovery that I was *not* holding the PA! We both took a deep breath as my heart almost jumped out of my mouth. There in my hand *was* the radio mike! There was dead silence on the Brooklyn North board. Then the radio meekly asked, "Unit with a message?"

"Uh, you can answer the radio for the rest of the night," I said, dropping the mike like a hot potato. Then we both got hysterical!

As the lone sector turned onto Eastern Parkway, it narrowly missed traffic. We saw the puffs of smoke from the lead car. The perps opened fire again.

"They're still firing. Where's the backup?" crackled the radio.

"Central, we need a bus here, Eastern, and Saratoga."

Central replied, "Is an officer down?"

"Just get us a bus!"

"EMS, we are one minute out, Central," Vinny said into his portable radio, monitoring the police frequency.

"EMS, please advise the condition," asked the police dispatcher with anxiety in her voice.

"Wilco."

Upon arriving, we found the two officers sitting in their car. There was a bullet hole through the windshield on the passenger's side.

"Oh Christ! One's hit!" Vinny yelled, as I brought the bus to a screeching halt. Vinny ran toward the officers as I got the equipment. Police cars pulled up, cops ran over to help. The pursuit of the perps was long forgotten.

"You stupid son of a bitch!" screamed the driver, still looking ahead, hands locked on the wheel.

"I'm sorry, John. I guess I got carried away."

"Are you hit? Where are you hit, man?" we screamed.

"He's gonna be *hit* in the fuckin' head once I control my temper," yelled the driver as the other cop stepped out. It seems they were taking fire from the perps when this officer pulled out his gun and returned fire. He took his time, aimed and shot. Unfortunately, he shot from inside the car, forgetting he had a windshield separating him from the bad guys.

As mentioned earlier, our ambulances broke down left and right, fire was not uncommon and the call volume continued to climb unabated.

With no support from Puzzle Palace (HQ) crews had to conduct their own triage of calls. One day we were assigned a "Cardiac," who was one of the regulars. The patient weighed just less than three hundred pounds, a true "quarter-pounder with cheese." She called at the same time, meeting us at the same corner, outside the same bar, on the same day each week. We got a little tired of this, but it was a living.

Lumbering to the side door of the unit, she waddled onto the crew bench. There she straightened out her loud floral print dress that wrapped her like the Goodyear blimp enveloping the gondola. Sweat poured from her forehead like a water fountain; I took a closer look at her. By all appearances, Helen looked like a larger black version of Tammy Baker. Bright red lipstick poorly smeared on large black lips almost gave them a clownish appearance. Dark stubble of hair could be observed above the upper lip as well as under her arms. Both eyes were masquerading as human under several uneven coats of eyeliner and all that. "Okay, Helen, give me your Medicaid and welfare cards."

The patient's fat, stubby fingers reached into the bad then gave me the cards.

"Thank you. Well, looks like you'll be getting a gift soon," I chuckled, attempting to get vital signs as my partner jotted down the information on the ACR. Once done he took out a hole puncher, popped two holes in the plastic cards before handing them back. I noted with satisfaction the cards were starting to look like Swiss cheese from all the holes punched. Other crews told certain "frequent flyers" that after they got enough holes in the cards, *they* received a gift. This hole punching procedure served two purposes. First, it was a way to identify who was abusing the system. Second, it would be the crews receiving a gift. The *gift* was the satisfaction that once the cards were ruined the patient would pay like hell in aggravation trying to get his or her welfare check. No cards, no check, no booze, no 911 call.

I was filling in the ACR when my partner called in a calm voice, "Hey, do you realize we're on fire?"

"No. Are you shitting me?"

"No, for real, smell." I looked through the hole into the crew compartment and, sure enough, there was the smell. Then a faint wisp of black smoke snaked its way toward the ceiling.

"I think we should start taking it into King's County. Don't you?"

"Yeah, let's get moving while we can." With the patient holding on to the straps, since they wouldn't reach around her leg much less her waist, the unit started moving with lights and siren.

"I had better let them know about this," my partner said, as the smoke became a bit thicker.

"You keep driving and pass me the mike. I'll tell them. Emergency. Emergency Thirty-three Charlie with an emergency."

"Thirty-three Charlie, what is your emergency?" the dispatcher asked, with annoyance in her voice. We probably interrupted her feeding cycle at the trough.

"Not much, just wanted to take a moment to inform you that we, Thirty-three Charlie, that's Charging Charlie, are on fire."

"What?"

"Yeah, sorry for disturbing you, but we are . . . <cough> . . . on <cough> . . . fire."

"Where are you? Pull over right now! Get out!"

"Negative, Central! Our first concern is patient care <cough>. We <cough> will be at the <cough> <cough> County in a few."

"Thirty-three Charlie? Thirty-three Charlie?"

"Do you mind <cough> if I smoke <cough> <cough> now?" my partner asked.

"Oh feel free <cough>. I'll brief Helen <cough>. Helen, as you can <cough> see, we are on fire <cough>. Don't be too upset or worry <cough>. Because it is your wish to go to the County again <cough> as one of our frequent flyers <cough>. We have decided <cough> not to stop and let you out."

Poor Helen was flailing around in the back of the bus like a massive blob of Jell-O, hanging on with both hands to the unattached seat strap. As the unit approached King's County, I started our 33 Chargin' Charlie emergency exit checklist.

"Helen, we hope to make it to King's County for your satisfaction. However, I must be honest with you. It doesn't look good. Now if this fire gets much worse, we may not be able to stop the vehicle with our brakes, and the cab may become an inferno. So I'm going to give you instructions for jumping."

Her eyes were now as wide as dinner plates and the fear was evident as she shook her head.

"Helen. Helen."

She looked.

"We want you to survive. We care about you. That's why we are risking our lives for you."

Her eyes were fixed in terror as I calmly continued.

"If I give the command to 'stand in the door,' you will pivot, turn from your seat, and stand like this." I demonstrated with my arms on each side of the door buck. "When I give the command 'Jump!' you will get out the door, away from the burning wreckage, aided with a gentle, but forceful shove from me. Once you hit the ground, you will hit five, well maybe for you, two points of contact."

Sweat ran like torrential rivers down her face, between layers of fat where a neck should have been. I continued my life-saving public service announcement.

"Upon exiting the burning ambulance, you will tuck in your arms and legs."

One look at her and I knew I'd have to modify that.

"Okay, I'll settle for your arms. Upon contact with terra firma, Mother Earth, you will hit with your feet first, rolling to your side. Here you will next make contact with your lower leg, upper thigh, well maybe in your case, it'll be one shot. Next, your butt and your back will make contact, coming to a safe halt. Is this understood?" I asked, accepting a blink from her petrified eyes as a yes. Glancing through the now thick smoke from the crew compartment, I checked how close we were to King's County. I knew as I turned back, black soot covered my sweat-covered face and white shirt.

"I think we just may make it, Helen!" I yelled over the pulsating, dying siren. We made the right turn into King's County, passing the garage; crews cheered as they coasted up the ramp, trailing black smoke from the burning bus and my partner's cigarette. Other crews met us with fire extinguishers as Helen was helped into the emergency room.

Helen never called 911 again. We saw her several months later at the hospital where a nurse said that Helen came in by taxi. Oh, the joy of healing people.

One day we, the County Mounties, had anywhere from three to four "Jumpers Down" jobs. It got so bad that the crews were giving points over the radio for their particular job.

"Mine was only an eight point five," crackled the radio. "He showed no form or grace and hit the building several times."

Another unit several minutes later: "I need ESU and medics for my jumper, Central."

"Condition?" inquired the dispatcher.

"A nine point five. She missed the sidewalk by four feet and is now impaled on a five-foot-tall iron fence."

"Alive?" asked the dispatcher.

"Yeah, doing the floppy chicken here. Put a rush on the medics."

Once the third job came across, with the unit announcing a "perfect ten," the floor lieutenant had enough and screamed at everyone. The remarks were quite graphic.

Another time, we backed up another Basic Life Support unit that responded to a "Man Pinned" at a construction site. The site was a building under reconstruction. The inside of the building was gutted, apartment by apartment. All the windows were out and new ones were soon to be put in. The job was reportedly on the fourth floor.

In the wrecked apartment, the EMTs called out to ask if anyone was hurt. No one answered. They called several times with no answer. After the final call, they heard a meek Haitian voice.

"Help. Please, help me," the voice said, coming from across the cluttered room. As one EMT tried to get the victim to say where he was, the other called for backup.

"I'm over here. Please move this stuff, hurry," came the trembling voice.

Meanwhile, we and a medic unit pulled up downstairs. As the two EMTs and the workers started to move the plywood sheets, broken beams, and furniture, the patient asked for them to hurry, explaining his leg was pinned by the old refrigerator.

The crew saw the refrigerator and worked at a fevered pitch. When they got to it, they couldn't see the patient. So they moved the refrigerator. There was a bloodcurdling scream. A plank snapped and dust flew everywhere. The crew thought the building was collapsing and joined in the chorus of screaming workers in running for the door. Then there was a deafening silence as the dust settled. Both crew members stood there looking at each other, when their radio crackled.

"Three Three David, your patient is down here with us," said the medic with a chuckle.

When our two heroes moved the refrigerator, which had pinned the patient to the wall, he was freed. By moving the refrigerator, they had managed to move the patient behind it, to an open space where the window used to be. He screamed as he exited the scene on the fourth floor and met us and the medics on the sidewalk next to the ambulance.

I learned from this experience that medics really appreciate it when you cut down the distance they have to carry their equipment *and* patient. Oh yeah, the patient survived.

One night, we had a job for a "Sick." When we entered the apartment, the daughter-in-law brought us into a dimly lit bedroom where we found an elderly, black woman. She was sitting in a chair, around which a sheet formed a sterile, safe cocoon isolating her from the physical world and human touch. Two dark eyes filled with a lifetime of shame, sorrow, and pain peered at us as we entered the poorly lit room.

"Hi, how can we help you, Mama?" I asked. She said she was sick. I asked for more light, explaining I would need to examine her and get vital signs. With the room now well lit, the woman lowered the sheet to the audible gasp of my partner.

The woman was covered with grotesque wart-like marks all over her body. Every half- inch on this person's face, neck, and eyelids was covered. The sight was more horrific than anything I had ever witnessed in combat or seen in any gothic film. Nauseated, I quickly deflected my train of thought to our higher goal as EMTs: to serve. This was not a leper, or a victim of smallpox, but a person first and foremost. Kneeling down beside her allowed me to focus on the task at hand as my fear evaporated. After I mentioned my ignorance of the disease that plagued her, she explained it was not contagious. It was indeed smallpox, contracted in Africa where she had lived most of her life. She came to King's County Hospital, hoping to find some relief for this affliction.

I looked at my partner, as I heard the cold elastic snap as he put on his sterile gloves. This annoyed me because she said she wasn't contagious. In a non-contagious situation, it seemed like the snap of the elastic was the sound of another artificial barrier being constructed, one she had endured from childhood. There are just too many damn barriers in this world and it's not natural.

I asked her if it would hurt her if I applied the blood pressure cuff and she answered no. So I reached over, *without* gloves, and did what I had to do including lung sounds. Her whole body was covered with this mask of ugliness, hiding the beauty of her humanity. What a tortured life she had endured. Placing her tenderly in our chair, my partner reminded me about my gloveless hands.

I smiled and held her hand, realizing how important flesh-to-flesh contact was to a soul condemned to a life in this organism we call the body. I believed anything, even something as small as holding someone's hand, done in an act of love, will protect you from any earthly physical contamination.

Anyone who has worked the streets realizes that a big part of our job is winning the confidence of patients. A lot of times, just holding their hands and listening was all that was needed, especially in this society of barriers. The result was universal.

We transported this treasure to King's County. As we removed her from the ambulance, she asked to be covered so no one would see her. Moving down the stark, sterile hall, we stopped momentarily as I spoke to a nurse. Two men were whispering and staring at her as she tried to withdraw deeper under the sheet.

"Hey! What the hell's the matter with you fuckin two idiots? This is a person just like you and me!" I yelled lividly as I took her hand from under the sheet and felt her squeeze it. They got the hint, and the nurse, realizing the urgency of the situation, moved her into the room.

Never let it be said that the police department was going to allow anyone to surpass them in education. One day we were standing by as two of New York's Finest (police officers) tried to talk down a would-be jumper from a window. All of us tried to talk the man back into the living room. But he wouldn't come in. The talking, reasoning and gentle persuasion went on for about forty-five minutes, until a new police sergeant showed up to take charge of the situation.

I was in mid-sentence with the distraught patient on the window ledge, when the sergeant stated, "Everyone out! I'll handle this. I just completed a course in psychology at John Jay College of Criminal Justice."

"Sarge, are you sure?" asked the anxious patrolman.

"Out, out," said the sergeant, as he ushered everyone out of the apartment. All stood listening to the sergeant's strategy, hoping to learn from his classes at this prestigious school.

"Okay, I'm Sergeant Jones. I understand you have a problem. So do I. My problem is my men and EMS have been tied up with you for more than an hour. You're wasting all our time and especially mine. So either jump or get in here now," demanded the sergeant. A lifetime passed. The door to the apartment opened and the sergeant stepped out. He was snow white.

He had demanded a decision of the patient and he got one. The guy jumped to his death. Oh well, back to the books.

It's always a special treat when working with both New York's Finest and New York's Bravest (firemen) together on a scene.

One cold, overcast, dreary day, we backed a medic unit for a "Cardiac Arrest" on the street. We pulled up simultaneously, seeing several firemen decked out in their fire garb, one holding a crowbar, talking to two cops. The streets were wet from fresh melted snow. A black male, about sixty years old, lay on the ground. His old, gray sports jacket was soaked, as he lay in a puddle. He was unkempt and undernourished. Next to his body was a brown bag with a broken liquor bottle of broken dreams.

"When did he go down? Anyone see it?" asked the medic, as we approached.

"Yeah, we saw him fall," said the fireman. We started to work on him as the police officers and firemen continued to talk.

"Oh, hey," interrupted the cop, as if having a second thought, "do me a favor and see if he has a wallet on him."

As the medic lay on his chest in the snow, intubating the man, I was doing the compressions and asked, "Why didn't you toss (search) him?"

"Oh, he's a skell and I didn't have gloves on me, so I figured I'd wait for you guys," he said, devoid of emotion.

As the intubation tube was being passed, the other medic was in the process of hooking up the monitor when I heard him mutter, "We'll get you for this, asshole."

The cop was lost in conversation with the others. They just stood there talking and enjoying themselves, oblivious to the drama that was taking place, as we fought for this man's life.

The monitor was put in place and the medic announced, "flat line," meaning there was no activity in the heart. I continued to do compressions, manually compressing the lifeless, motionless heart to circulate blood to the brain and kidneys.

My knees hurt as I kneeled in the cold water on the cracked concrete, and my lower back throbbed in spasmodic pain as I bent over the patient. My partner bagged the patient with the BVM via the intubation tube at the patient's head, providing life-saving oxygen to the breathless man.

The medics gave medications, first down the tube, and then into the IV. They hoped the medications would start the heart of this man. All that was needed was one cell in the heart to start. In this wonder we call the center of love, the heart, if one cell fires, the others will start their Dance of Life automatically. But here on this overcast day, nothing was happening.

"Hey look," I said as the monitor came alive with another rhythm.

"It's v-fib." (Instead of firing in sequence, the heart cells start firing at once—totally ineffective, like Jell-O.)

Both experienced medics realized it was only chemically induced from the potent drugs. They knew there was little hope for this man but they also knew it was payback time. For the man's sake and the crews' peace of mind, they were about to take revenge on both the police and firemen for not doing anything to help this "skell" the crews treasured so dearly.

As the county medic grabbed for the paddles on the monitor, he winked at us as he placed them on the old man's naked chest.

"Hey, you guys," his partner called to the cops and firemen. "My partner is going to shock this guy. As you can see, you guys are standing on a wet street and electricity travels through water. So when you hear me say 'three' I want you to jump, so you are not in the water when he defibrillates the guy. Got it?"

All parties watched with concern, listening for the count. One fireman looked down at his rubberized boots in the water.

"Hey!" yelled the medic, "are you daydreaming? This will kill you."

"No, I'm listening," the fireman said.

His buddies told him, "Pay attention, brother. Remember, at the count of three."

"Ready?" asked the medic.

"Yeah, three, we're ready," came the chorus. The medic turned to his partner and both had devious smirks on their faces. The medic called, "I'm clear, one. You're clear, two. Everybody's clear, three. JUMP!"

The medic depressed the twin red buttons, sending a massive jolt of energy through the patient's body. This caused his body to jump up, along with the horrified cops and firemen. It was as if the old man knew that the medics were having these men make idiots out of themselves for his benefit and he wanted to get one last look.

The medics and EMTs broke up as they searched for a pulse on the old man. The seasoned medic realized none would be found, but also realized the old man had given his approval to the crews to attempt to pay back the Finest and Bravest for their lack of respect for this "skell." I learned the police are New York's Finest, the firemen, New York's Bravest. But the crews of EMS are still New York's Smartest.

It was interesting that I never knew whom I might meet, under what conditions.

One day, we were given an EDP (Extremely Disturbed Person) or "Every Day Person" to the crews. We pulled up to the private house and entered. The police led the way down a hallway with the living room. In the living room sat several male blacks enjoying the football game on TV. We heard one gentleman say, without breaking his stare from the game like the rest, "Marvin is upstairs."

The woman who was directing us said, "He's blind, holding a four-foot cross of Jesus, going crazy smashing stuff." She then turned and walked back into the kitchen.

We got this job a few weeks after Eleanor Bumpers was shot dead by ESU of the police department. She had been an older, black woman, who reportedly attempted to attack the cops with a knife.

The ESU cop looked at me, the strain showing on his face, and remarked, "Great, just what I fuckin' need. I can see it now on the front page of the *New York Post*, 'Cops kill a blind, black man while he was holding a giant cross of Jesus.'"

I laughed and so did he. As it turned out, we talked Marvin into lowering the cross long enough for us to overpower him without hurting him.

On another call, we entered an apartment to find a black female about twenty years old, walking around in a daze in the kitchen. She was extremely thin, black hair unkempt, and wearing an open housecoat. She was definitely not with the program. She pointed to the stove and then said, "Plane, plane," pointing skyward.

"What the hell is she talking about?" asked a cop.

"Perhaps she means the stove will blow up and we'll all meet a plane in the sky," his partner said.

The door to the hallway was open and as the cops searched the kitchen, three black men looked in.

"Do you know this woman?" I asked.

"No, we've never seen her," came the reply.

"Do you know what she's saying?" we asked, figuring perhaps they recognized the language she was now speaking.

"Hell, man, we're Americans," came the curt remark.

"Fine, then take a walk," the cops said.

As the search continued, a black male walked into the apartment, picked up the mail on the table, opened it, and started reading it, ignoring all around him. The woman was on her knees, imploring him. We all stopped what we were doing and just stared. Finally the cop said, "Hey, what the hell are you doing?"

"I'm reading my mail," he said, without looking up. The cop reached over and ripped the mail from the man's hand, forcing some eye contact.

"I'll ask you again, who are you?"

With burning anger in his eyes, the five-foot-two man responded with his name.

"And who is she?"

"She is my subject."

"Excuse me?" the flabbergasted cop asked.

"She is my subject. She has come from my native land in Africa to visit and worship me."

"And who are you?"

"I am her king."

"And what are you doing here in America?"

"I drive a cab."

"Only in America," I said, as we started to laugh.

It turned out that the king had female subjects visit him. Evidently, this one did not appreciate the royal treatment she was receiving, so he was banishing her with the threat of passing word back to her family, thus dishonor. This sent her over the edge.

We packaged the *subject* into the chair and restrained her, as she thrashed, screaming not to be taken away from her king.

As we left the apartment, the king stood erect, reading mail, and ignoring the tearful pleas of his subject. Like I said, only in America!

Someone called in a "Cop Shot" at a "House of Ill Repute" on Coney Island Avenue. The cops as well as we responded. Up the stairs everybody trudged. The cops banged on the iron mesh gate and a large bouncer opened it. He was more than three hundred pounds of pure Italian muscle, with a large bulldog face, accentuated by a six-inch scar across his right cheek. The cops emptied everyone out of the rooms. It really hadn't been a busy night for the girls and most were sitting on the couch in various modes of undress, along with the one John.

The madam and her bouncer watched as the cops went from room to room. The madam asked if we would like something to drink, explaining her rival was doing this, and proceeded to give the officers information. The girls were a splendid and healthy lot as opposed to some of the "ladies" we had seen. One of the girls, who was Italian, about five-foot-four, approached us.

"Would you check my heart, please?" she asked my new partner in a purring sound from her luscious, pursed red lips.

The cops looked at the barefoot goddess, as he turned beet red and stuttered, "No, I . . . I . . . can, can't do that."

Her playful, green eyes sparkled, "Oh." She turned ever so gently, as if on an unseen wisp of air, allowing her breasts to innocently brush his chest, the electric charge forcing him to jump back. As she swirled, the blue chiffon nightgown glided in sync with rich jet-black hair, carrying the youthful scent of unseen promises. She looked up into my eyes.

"Would you check my heart?"

"Certainly, I will," I responded in a soft, knowing voice. Without breaking eye contact with her, reaching over, I grabbed my partner's stethoscope. Sensually, she reached to drop the nightgown to expose her "heart." I placed my hands tenderly over hers, feeling the heat generated from her chest. The room was still. My partner was in shock, frozen in place. The cops maneuvered to get a ringside seat to view her beautiful "heart."

Still entranced, never ending eye contact with the girl, my hands still on hers, I whispered, "A lady like you deserves to have her heart checked, but in private."

You could hear the moans of disgust, as she smiled with the excitement of a child who was just given a precious gift. Holding my hand, she led me into the empty room. As I closed the door, I smiled at a shocked and sad group. The madam winked her approval as I smiled, closing the door. Privacy, confidentiality, and public relations are important. Hey, trust me! Oh and yes, she did have a *beautiful heart*, all *two of them!*

It was another typical autumn day in Brooklyn. The holidays would soon be here, as would the out-of-court settlements from "injuries" received from a problem with the elevator or the infamous "falling ceiling."

Thus we received a call for a "Falling Ceiling" in an apartment building. On the scene, we found a female Haitian sitting at a kitchen table, her head strategically resting on her folded arms on a table alive with roaches. We were informed there was a chunk of ceiling in the tub, but the girlfriend said it happened in the bedroom, according to the cop filling us in. They wanted to go to the hospital to start the paper trail of "pain and suffering," he said, trying not to laugh.

I checked her out and found nothing except a light layer of white powder on the top of her black greasy hair. There was no trauma except what was caused by *low-velocity dust*. Had it been high-velocity dust, it would have at least made it to her scalp. I needed to ask some questions, so the cop called her friend who was in the bedroom, getting the patient's coat ready.

"Yo, Loony, come out here."

"Ah, come on," I said, chuckling, "we both know what the deal is, but there's no point in insulting her."

"Insult? Hell, watch this," the Haitian interpreter came out to the kitchen. "Would you please show this fine EMT your passport." Sure enough, it read Loony Lunatic. We tried not to laugh and couldn't wait to get to King's County to introduce this person to the nurse. Oh and yes, after being informed to knock the bullshit dramatics off, the patient walked to the bus without incident.

At the County, one of the nurses did take my report. As she spoke to Loony, I stood waiting for her to sign my ACR. Well, she was in no hurry, so I reached in my pocket into a box of raisins I was eating. With the flick of a finger I shot a large raisin across her desk. Startled, she jumped as I slammed the moving raisin with my hand. Then picked it up, examined it and ate it. The old nurse looked horrified at me. "What? It's good protein!" With this, she signed the ACR. "I could kiss you," I said, stepping toward her. She ran into the hallways, screaming about "That crazy white boy is eating roaches!"

Interesting names are just one of the fun things I encountered on the job. The other was the ghetto mentality. One time we responded to a call for a child who was sick. Getting off the elevator, we turned the corner in the welfare hotel, as the woman holding the child coughed. Her friend quickly put out the cigarette lighter, placed it behind her back, dropping it to the floor as she turned. The mother held up a thermometer and said, "Look. It's very hot." Sure was; the kid would have been dead if it were an accurate temperature.

You play the part by asking, "Was this a rectal temperature?"

"It sure was."

Of course it's all bullshit, since she was holding a child fully clothed. We took them down to the bus and started filling out the ACR, since the walls and floor were moving with roaches.

We asked the child's name and were told, "Feemally Jones."

"And how do we spell Feemally?" my partner asked.

With indignation, the mother passed us the identification papers; it read, "Female Jones." You cannot make this stuff up. Working the streets you know it's all true.

In New York, the melting pot of the world, there can be a problem with language.

"Excuse me, sir," I asked one nasty drunk. "Have you been the victim of a drowning within the last twenty-four hours?"

"No."

"Okay. How about the victim of a homicide within the last twelve hours?"

"No, man."

"Very good, sir. One last question then. Are you a *Homo sapiens*?"

"Yo, mother fucker! I likes women, not men."

"Thank you, sir."

In the County area of Brooklyn, I delivered my share of infants. I counted just under twenty deliveries, including three sets of twins.

Once, we had a twelve-year-old Hispanic female with "Abdominal Pains." The mother got insulted and yelled at us when I asked the daughter how long she had been pregnant. It was a losing battle, so we took her down in the chair. The kid wouldn't answer the questions and the mother yelled, "Not my child. How dare you insult us. I'll have your job."

In the back of the bus, the daughter lay on the stretcher, not saying anything, and the mother glared at me. Well, guess what? The baby had it with both of them and started coming out.

"Pull over, we'll do it here," I said to my partner. He came to the back and climbed in, and we ignored the mother. As we delivered the baby, there was a thump on the floor. Good old "I'm going to have your job. Not my daughter" hit the floor. Once revived and at the hospital, this new grandmother never even said thanks. Not all deliveries go this well.

A friend of mine, also named Jim, told me of this experience years ago when we worked together at the County. The last I heard, Jimmy was doing well in NYPD. Ah yes, another EMS success story! His unit responded to a "Pregnant Female." They pulled up to the address and noted with relief that the apartment was on the first floor. They entered the dilapidated tenement and stood in silence, noting they had stepped into a different world. A woman answered the door, invited them in, and sat down on a blue satin couch.

"Don't worry about the carpet, gentlemen. Please come in," she said with a warm Caribbean smile and accent.

The patient was a thirty-three-year-old professional Jamaican. The way she gracefully sat, eloquent speech, and her plain, but elegant, dress bestowed grace on a tired crew.

"How might we help you, mama?"

"Sir, as you can see I am pregnant and felt I needed your assistance to get to the hospital."

As one crew member did the vital signs, the other asked her medical history as he sat at a sculptured wooden dining room table, on a lush carpet.

"Okay, mama, we're ready. Please have a seat in our chair."

"Oh please, I'd rather walk. You men look tired."

"We are mama, but not too tired to carry you. Besides, it's the right thing to do and we haven't dropped anyone all day," the EMT said with a smile.

"Okay then," she said, standing up and adjusting her light blue patterned dress. Once erect, she let out a surprising scream and grabbed her stomach. Then Jim grabbed her as she fell writhing to the floor.

"Go get the stretcher fast," he directed his partner who ran out the door.

"It's coming! It's coming," she screamed.

"It's okay. It's okay. Look at me. Work on your breathing. I'm here, don't worry."

"God, it hurts so bad," she cried, as she clawed his hand.

"Mama, I'm going to have to examine you, so please let go of my hand." *Hell,* he thought, *no big deal. She said it was her first, so we'll have plenty of time. Plus, I've delivered enough.*

After removing her skirt and slip, she started to pull her legs up to her stomach as she started to sob, "It's coming, God."

"Don't worry. I'm here. Do you know how many kids me and my partner have—" He never had time to finish the sentence. As he removed her lace panties, he was greeted with two feet

"Oh shit," he muttered. His partner walked through the door with the stretcher, turned and heard Jim yell, "Breech birth!" Grabbing his radio, he called for a medic unit. Jim turned back to face the patient and he saw four feet!

"Holy shit," he yelled, as he inserted his fingers into her vagina to keep the airway open for the kids.

"Wha . . . is that?" his partner asked, with a confused look on his face.

"We need help and fast. Where the fuck are the medics?"

"None available, Central said."

"Okay, we have to think."

"The cops are sitting in their car." They were there as usual, behind the bus, waiting for us to bring out the patient and information to them. "I'll get them," the partner said as he ran outside to enlist the help of the cops, while Jim became acquainted with his new friend.

The contractions came and went, each time building in intensity and agony. Suddenly, another typhoon of spasms hit. Jim fought to keep his fingers in her vagina as she squeezed, crushed, and scratched his other hand with her long fingernails. All the time, he tried to keep her from rolling on the floor as her body jerked spasmodically in uncontrolled convulsions. Jim continued to talk to her through the bloodcurdling screams.

"Get it out. Take it out," she shrieked, until the spasm crested and began to recede. Then her body relaxed briefly. He adjusted his fingers in her vagina, got circulation back in his other hand, said a silent prayer for help, and cursed the medics they needed so badly.

He could feel his own fear bubbling under the surface, but he could not show it to the patient, who depended on him. Sweat poured from him, as he tasted the salt, making him even more thirsty.

With the help of the two cops—one held her hands, the other the waist—they lifted her onto the stretcher. Jim told the cop to sit in the captain's chair at her head and not to let go of her arms. His partner informed him that medics were now free.

"Screw them. Let's get the fuck out of Dodge!"

"You got it, Tonto. I'll call ahead to King's County," his partner said, as he closed the rear doors. Although it had been rather cool, sweat now ran down his shirt like Niagara Falls. The bus hurtled through the streets with its siren wailing, a plea to move out of the way for the precious cargo. As Jim turned to fling some salty sweat from his eyes, he saw the police car. It was right behind, lights flashing, siren wailing. A passenger car almost hit the police car!

Assholes! When will people learn? he thought. Then it happened. The mother of all spasms brutally erupted.

"Get it out," she frantically screamed, violently twisting as she now fought with galactic strength to break free from the cop's grip. "Now!"

At that moment, the bus hit a pothole and the cop lost his grip. The woman broke the stretcher strap across her chest. With her free hands, she smacked Jim, who was kneeling. Knocked off balance by the pothole, he went crashing to the floor. In a split second, he heard a primordial scream escape his lips, "No!" Reaching between her legs, grabbing the four legs in one herculean move, she pulled, resulting in an explosive projection of the children from her vagina. Suddenly, as she looked down in horror, an ungodly fear contorted her once elegant face. She attempted to scream as her swollen eyes met Jim's, but she passed out

Jim checked the mother for a pulse and then repositioned her. Since her respirations were good, he placed an oxygen mask on her then checked for copious bleeding. Next, he moved to her babies. Each baby had one head, two arms and two legs. But now he understood her unspoken terror.

The babies were Siamese twins, joined at the chest. The cop gagged, recoiling at the sight, as Jim yelled at him to open the multi-trauma and wet it. He tenderly cleaned the babies, sick to his stomach, wondering what would become of them. Their breathing was fine. Except for the fact they were joined and they looked underweight, they appeared normal in all other respects. He turned, spit on his index finger, and made a sign of the cross on each head, asking God's blessing on them.

He moved to the mother as the cop cried, "I'm sorry, so sorry. I couldn't hold her." There was nothing to say. The siren went off as the bus made the familiar right turn and started going up the ramp. The staff and two other EMS crews were there to assist. The children died about a week later.

It was New Year's Eve in Brooklyn and we were ready for the coming trauma. As we pulled out of King's County, we stopped for coffee. I sat sipping my coffee while my partner went to get a chicken dinner. All at once, I heard a thud as a livery cab rear-ended a car stopped at the light. There was minimal damage. The drivers got out and screamed at each other. I continued to sip my coffee until the driver of the lead car saw the bus (ambulance) and came over. I picked up the radio to report the flag down for the accident and ask for the police to do the paperwork.

As I talked to the dispatcher, the driver ran up.

"Yeah, Central, the location is Flatbush and Church. No, we are not involved in the collision."

All of a sudden, the guy yelled, "Don't say you are not involved."

People stopped to watch this black man ask help from a white EMT, who said he did not want to get involved. Some in this community look for trouble at the drop of a hat. Halfway through my conversation with the dispatcher, I told the guy, "Shut the fuck up and get over to your car, asshole." He did and I finished my conversation with the dispatcher. I got out and walked over to look at the minor bullshit. "Okay, since both of you are fine, just pull your vehicles over to the side and start exchanging your information. The cops will be here when they can."

One thing I learned on the street was to read a situation. I heard my little voice tell me that the second driver was going to split. As the first guy pulled over, the second guy flew out and I dove onto the hood of the first car to avoid a high-speed rundown feeling.

The moron, instead of going straight, turned onto Church Avenue and wound up stopping in traffic. Remember what your mama said about always locking all your doors? Well, I bolted off the hood of the vehicle and sprinted after the car. As I approached, a sector from the

Sixty-seventh Precinct came from the opposite direction on Church Avenue and saw me. At first they thought I was getting a lift from a friend, until they saw my equipment belt. I ran up alongside the car, which now was only moving at about three miles an hour.

The driver, a Haitian in his thirties, looked in his driver's side mirror as he escaped. I jumped in and caught his face with my right fist, as he turned to see the intruder. With his nose broken and bleeding, I followed up with another shot, breaking his lip. Both of his hands came up to protect his face, as I slammed the car into park. The impact, even at a low speed, sent me crashing into the dash. Grabbing the keys, I killed the engine. The cops pulled abreast of us, threw on their lights, and jumped out.

A crowd formed and was being agitated by this overweight ghetto beast. The cops grabbed the guy, who resisted arrest and was trying to incite the still forming crowd. Once he was cuffed, they unceremoniously threw his ass into the back of the car. One cop pulled the guy's car over and locked it.

A bimbo screamed, "I saw it! He hit the brother for no reason. The white medic tried to rob him."

I told the cops we'd meet at the Sixty-seventh Precinct. They wanted to get out of the area fast, which is always the best way to diffuse the situation. But they were worried about me.

"Go ahead, I'll be fine," I told them as they pulled down the street. As I walked back to the bus, she followed me on the sidewalk so I got into her ugly, fat face. Looking into her hate-filled eyes, I screamed at the top of my lungs, "Yo, shut the fuck up, ho (whore)! Or you'll get worse. And do something about your fuckin' breath!"

People started to laugh. The situation was defused with the aid of laughter. The cops saw I was in the unit safely and sped the perp out of the area. I picked up the radio as my partner got in with his dinner.

"32 America."

"32 America," responded the dispatcher.

"32 America with one under. Will be going to the Sixty-seventh Precinct for the paperwork."

"I'm afraid to even ask. Just give me a land line when you get there."

Later that evening we received a call for a "Man Under" in the subway. We grabbed our gear as we pulled up to the most depressing subway station in the world. The transit cops, along with the ESU, were on the scene.

"You have two guys hit by a train about two hundred feet inside the tunnel. Follow us." We went into the hole, as we call a subway job. We walked along a garbage-littered, depressingly lit platform to the end. The smell of human feces and urine surrounded us even before we climbed off the platform.

On the track level, we walked into a dark abyss, guided by the cop's mag light.

"If a train should come, drop your gear, find and hug one of these cutouts," he said. We passed several cutouts, but he neglected to say what we all knew. If a train came, at full speed, it would suck us out of the cutout, killing us *if* we were *lucky.*

Onward we walked, into the bowels of the endless tunnel. I slipped several times in the polluted water, scratching and swatting at the orbiting ferocious fleas and mites. We stopped for a moment to adjust our equipment and I felt something on my foot. I flashed my mag to see a rat parked on my boot

"Shit," I yelled, flipping the rodent off. The heat in this eternal nocturnal world of squalor was morbidly suffocating. Yet here, too, was a city within a city. People lived here. People few saw and even less cared about. It almost became a hardship to breathe in the oppressive stench as a phalanx of orbiting livestock eagerly competed with stifling humid air to enter my nostrils. I saw a light and prayed it wasn't a train. I didn't feel the breeze in the tunnel, only the low hum coming from the third rail, so I figured we were safe.

Two jobs make me leery: subway and highway. Through the years and many train jobs, transit police always have told us, "The power's off."

I have always asked, "Well, if this is so, how come the car lights are still on?" Never have received an answer.

As we trudged closer, I saw a cop holding his light over an elderly black man writhing in pain on the side of the track. He lay in a puddle of water on his right side, holding his right leg. We could see the gravity of the situation. His right leg was cut off about six inches above his knee. The left foot sat in the shoe about fifteen feet from him and rodents were already gnawing at it. They didn't flinch even when the lights were shined on them. The cop saved his leg by pulling it closer and actually holding it upright against the guy's back

"We need medics," my partner said.

"No shit, Sherlock. Let's get to work on him until they get here." We squatted in the filth, treating the mangled wounds with trauma dressings and cling. The good news was the heat of the amputation had seared the wounds closed, but part of his femur, the long bone in the upper leg, showed. It protruded about four inches from the burned flesh, which had shriveled the leg, exposing the bone. We tried to comfort him the best we could. As the man moved, his amputated leg resting behind him fell on him and he screamed

"We have to get that on ice," I said, trying to divert the guy's attention. It worked.

"Can you save it, doc?" the guy asked.

"We're gonna try," I said, looking at the cop. Both of us realized it probably couldn't be saved.

"There's a bar on the corner, I'll go for some ice."

"Okay, but don't get lost or drunk," I said. The cop took off with the guy's leg wrapped with a multi-trauma dressing on the exposed end. We heard the medics coming and we saw a light approaching from the other end.

"Fuck," I said, reaching over and tapping my partner.

"Oh shit," he said, as the medics showed up and we felt the breeze of doom. The cop was on the radio, yelling. The old man looked at us.

"Sucks to be me, son. Why don't you youngsters get the hell out of here?"

"What, and leave you?" the medic said, getting an IV set.

"Look, I've lived here all my life."

He was cut short as I asked, "Where?"

"Here. You're Irish, aren't you?"

"Yeah, but not a black Irishman." He exploded in laughter, reaching up and squeezing my hand. I've always believed if the patient laughs, he'll do fine. If not, I worry.

"I've lived here in these tunnels."

The cop tapped the medic. "These assholes keep saying the power's off, but those fuckin' lights are still on. We have to move."

"Where?" the female medic asked.

If we moved, it would be to save ourselves in the cutouts. The patient would never make it.

"Go on," the old guy said, resigned to his fate. The female looked at her partner, then at us. The years on the street showed in her tired eyes. But so did the compassion of her heart. The cop was getting jittery.

"My partner is out there looking for this asshole's friend."

"Hey," said the male medic, "we are not leaving anyone, understand?" It was a statement, not a question.

"If you want to hit the cutout, no big deal, honestly, we'll understand," I said. The old man squeezed the medic's hand as he looked and smiled. The breeze of death was getting stronger, now hitting us just short of typhoon wind. Suddenly we saw a smaller light bouncing like a firefly in front of the bigger one. It was the cop's partner. He was slipping and sliding in the center of the tracks, heading our way

"Hey, I found the other guy! I found the other guy!" When the black cop got to us, he was huffing and puffing. "There must be a fuckin' dead spot out there. I could hear you but I knew you couldn't hear me," he said to his partner.

"A fuckin' Jesse Owens you're certainly not," said his partner, and we all started laughing. The stark terror hit when we heard a blast of the train's whistle.

"Holy shit," we shouted in unison, as it scared the hell out of us all.

"Got you, white boys," he paused, catching his breath, seeing the female medic, "and girls. Scared, huh?" said the cop with a big smile on his face. "I had them stop."

"Fuck you, Jesse," was all his partner could say.

"Listen, why don't you show me where this guy's friend is," I suggested.

"Thanks," said the medic, as they were still checking the guy out. I grabbed my tech bag and mag light and off we went.

"He was moaning, on the side with a broken leg. I moved him up to a pillar and sat him up as I ran to stop the train," the cop told me. When we got to the scene, he said, "Watch his leg." He gingerly attempted to hold it in place as I stepped next to the guy. The lights from the stopped train were blindly cutting through the eternal darkness. In the light I could see the vermin darting back and forth. Above the lights I could see the engineer and passengers peering into our darkness. The patient was indeed sitting where the cop helped place him.

"Was this guy talking to you?" I asked.

"Yeah. He was screaming about the pain. But when I felt the breeze and saw the light appear, I knew I had to stop the train or we would all be killed. So I moved him to safety as best I could. He even told me his name was Payday."

"Before he was moved, right?"

"Yeah." Then it struck him, as he knelt in the mixture of water, grease and God knows what, holding the guy's leg. The young man was dead. His neck was snapped. I stood over the cop as he started to cry. The train silhouetted us in this darkened hell some call home. I reached over and squatted down, placing an arm around the cop and Payday. After what seemed to be an eternity, we walked back to the platform to see if we could help with the first patient.

The fire department had showed up, another BLS unit, and a patrol boss. The patient was in the back of the medic bus.

"Sir, I'm sorry to have to tell you. Payday is dead," I said, standing outside the bus. He looked up to the ceiling as tears rolled down his cheeks.

"Hey, you're not leaving me now, are you? It's New Year's Eve," the old man called, as the medic adjusted the IV.

"Yeah, I guess so."

"Hey, why don't you hop in? I may need a hand," said the medic. The backup EMTs and fire removed Payday.

"Here's your leg," said the cop. He did indeed have it wrapped in plastic and ice from the bar across the street.

"Did the guy give you a hard time?" asked the medic.

"Yeah, until I unwrapped it on the fuckin' bar. All I saw were assholes and elbows. The bartender was a cool dude from Vietnam."

"So, you had a beer while safeguarding the leg?" I asked with a smile.

"You're damn right, several."

We transported to Bellevue Hospital trauma and replant center. En route, the patient looked at me. His eyes showed yellow from jaundice. He was a light-skinned black man with gray whiskers, dark, cracked lips, and gray matted hair. Blotches of grease covered parts of his head and hands. His hands were like large gloves, dry with cracks in them. His tattered, corduroy shirt had been cut away during his physical exam. A faded brown belt held up what was left of his pants. With two IVs in his arm, he attempted to reach us.

"Doc, am I going to make it?" The medic looked at me.

"Well, you sure as shit won't be break dancing tonight. But yeah, you'll do fine," I said, reaching for his hand. He and the medic were hysterical.

"You sure are an Irishman," he said, grabbing our hands. With the howling in the back, the female medic called, "Is everything okay?"

"It couldn't be better," responded her partner.

For me, King's County was the place to work. EMS was still relatively small, more like an extended family. The hospital was run by Dr. Clark, who tried to get the funding for the largest facility in the United States that dealt with third world diseases. People came from all over the world to be treated. Since these people were from third world nations, the majority was not white. Thus there was a problem with funding. America, the greatest country in the world, is plagued with color issues. But there were saints like Dr. Clark, Dr. Agular of the County, and Dr. Trowers in Harlem.

THREE

Stress Free One Oh Zee

After three years as an EMT and being tutored by legendary medics, I finally went to the EMS Paramedic Program at Ft. Totten, wanting to provide a higher level of care to my patients. Because of a learning disorder, it would take me two programs to complete what others had done in one. Instructors Lori Santo (Mom), and Dave Russell were the two who saw something in me and made room for me. Thus I graduated with Class 8, in 1988. After filling several slots on vacation relief, I finally got a unit: 10Z. I named the unit Stress Free One Oh Zee. We were deployed as a tactical unit wherever needed. We were in a dynamic mode and able to shift locations. This included the five boroughs to assist with call volumes. One of the problems we encountered was not deployments, but dispatches. We came out of Bellevue Hospital at Twenty-eighth Street and First Avenue in Manhattan at 6:00 P.M.

On more than one occasion, they gave us a "Cardiac Arrest" at Vermilyea Avenue with a cross of 207th Street. We dealt with rush-hour traffic in midtown Manhattan, traveling to a "Cardiac Arrest" close to two hundred blocks away. Within four minutes the brain starts to deteriorate. Dispatch gave us a hard time if we asked for a backup. One of their classic responses was, "You're solo." Or the totally brainless statement, "You're computer recommended." This was, of course, after the dispatcher called the lieutenant telling him the tour commander wanted us rushed into service. Once told we were in service, the dispatcher would move us over on the computer into our area uptown. Needless to say, this is not about nor ever was about patient care requirements. It was about inept idiots conning the public.

In those days, we were not allowed on certain parts of FDR Drive because of the weight of the vehicles. There was an order as such. The chiefs were fast to have a lieutenant write you up for this infraction. Most people left within three to four years. Stress Free would boldly go where no other unit went before

We had a reputation of volunteering to back up any Basic unit. This tradition of Stress Free started before I became a medic. Although I named the unit, there were three legends that came before me. These were bright shining lights of hope. As an EMT, I definitely looked up to them for their knowledge, esprit de corps, and their trademark.

Paramedics John McFarlin, Jim Kelly and Don Boyce responded to any unit calling for medics. It did not matter what was the weather—rain, sleet, snow, heat wave—or time of day. These guys stepped out of Ten Zebra wearing long-sleeve, spotless white shirts, ties, ironed green pants, and spit-shined black shoes. With shields shining on their chests, stethoscopes around their necks, and the ever-ready smile, their mere presence brought a sense of professionalism and healing. Their dedication and excellence have never been matched.

One of my partners was "Fat Joe." This clown gave medicine by color, not the color on the label of the bottle, but the color of the person he was serving. Blacks didn't get anything. Hispanics might get oxygen. Those who were white and could write attaboy letters to the EMS god got the world, whether they needed it or not. He was fond of pointing out that his father was a retired Supreme Court judge.

My first experience with him was when we got a call for an "Unconscious." An elderly black woman led us and our backup crew of EMTs through a well-kept apartment, directing us into the living room. The woman's sixty-one-year-old sister lay on the couch. She was conscious and stated, "I'm going to die."

Joe, who was teching, looked at her, "Okay. If you don't want to go to the hospital, just sign the paper and we'll leave." The horrified crew looked at me as he went for his pen. The sister, who had years of suffering etched on her face, stood in silence.

"Okay, medical consultation," I said, firmly grabbing Fat Joe's shoulder, and directed him toward our better sides. "We are going to work her and then take her to the hospital."

"I'm the senior paramedic and I think . . ."

Before he could finish his proclamation, I shot him a look that registered like a five-hundred-pound smart bomb on a dumb target. I knelt down and spoke to the woman on the couch, explaining our plan. That night, we worked up the lady and transported her to the hospital. She was indeed having a heart attack.

Another time, we were deployed to Spanish Harlem where Fat Joe got nosebleeds. He loved midtown with its money and influential people.

We were in Spanish Harlem when an ESU (Police Emergency Service Unit) encountered their worst nightmare. A raid was made on a known drug location. The police started by announcing themselves. These guys always have manners. When the gentleman in question did not respond in kind, the police started beating down the door. The "dealer" decided to hide the coke by ingesting it.

The cops broke the door, announced themselves again, and entered to find the dealer sitting in the kitchen. With their guns drawn, they told him to stand so they could cuff him. A short skirmish erupted while they put the cuffs on him, but he was overpowered. They sat him on a chair, but he fell to the floor. Prisoners often pull this. But he was down for good, in cardiac arrest!

My former unit, 14B from Metropolitan, responded. They found the guy in arrest and started working on him. They were told there were no medics, so they carried him down five flights and loaded him into the bus. We heard the call and put ourselves on it. At the same time another medic unit from Roosevelt Hospital started to respond. The race was on.

I pulled up to the Roosevelt unit, grabbed the gear, and ran for the Basic bus. Roosevelt pulled up and one of their medics hopped in the back. I tubed the patient, got him on a monitor, gave him the first round of drugs, and started looking for the line. Fat Joe waddled in. He liked to remind me, and anyone else within earshot, that he was the "*senior medic*" on the scene. Title talk really endeared him to me.

Fat Joe sat, shouting commands. Mind you, not doing anything, just shouting. I had a hard time gaining IV access on the guy and the Roosevelt medic asked to try.

"Oh no," said Fat Joe, "This is an EMS job."

The medic looked at me. "Fuck him. Everybody goes for it." The medic from Roosevelt got the line. Once he got the flashback and knew he was in, I passed him the IV and the second round of drugs. Meanwhile, Fat Joe kept up his tirade from his ceremonial position on the bench, never lifting a hand to help. Finally, I had had enough of listening to Fat Joe, so I thanked the other unit, got out and walked back to Stress Free.

We pulled into Saint Luke's Hospital and offloaded the dead guy, who had gone to cocaine heaven. As I stood talking with the EMTs, Fat Joe came up in a huff.

"I'm the senior medic here," he yelled, as he stuck his fat finger into my chest

The next thing I heard was a voice crying, "I've been assaulted! I've been assaulted!" It was coming from what appeared to be a beached whale lying on the floor.

"So you're hurt, you worthless piece of shit? Want to go to a hospital? If you're not on your feet in thirty seconds, I'll place your fat useless ass on a long board and take you to Harlem," I said. After a few attempts he got up and tried to win the crew, not realizing it was my old unit.

"You saw what happened, right? He assaulted me."

The EMT responded, "Yeah, we saw what happened. You pushed Jim, then tripped. Want to go to Harlem?" Fat Joe went inside and called Bellevue reporting I, of all people, assaulted him, when I was only checking for a backbone via his stomach. I never found his backbone.

He came out of the ER lividly proclaiming, "We are ten-sixty-two, Out of Service, back to Bellevue where I will press charges!"

"Okay," I responded, as I turned the radio knob to an oldies channel.

When we arrived at Bellevue, he had to waddle in fast to talk to the lieutenant on duty. I sat listening to a song, waiting for it to finish, and then followed him inside. EMT and friend, Sid Lewis, sat outside. Sid had worked with me at King's County.

"What did you do to poor Fat Joe?" he asked with a smile.

"Me? What are you talking about, Sid?"

"Listen, he came waddling by me, screaming for the lieutenant, holding his stomach. You come in here singing with a smile on your face. I know you did something." I just smiled and started to enter the door, when Fat Joe came out, holding his stomach.

"Follow me! The lieutenant is in the medic room."

"Yes, oh fat senior medic," I said, looking at Sid smiling, and started to whistle again.

Fat Joe explained his problem to Lieutenant Freddie Marine.

"He assaulted me."

"Prove it," I said. Freddie looked at me and I noted a smile under his gray handlebar mustache.

"Sir, the crew of Four Boy will give you statements that Fat Boy here assaulted me, then tripped," I said in a non-confrontational manner, cranking Fat Joe even more.

"That's a lie!"

"Are you saying that three members of the service are liars?" Freddie asked.

"Uh no," Fat Joe quietly answered. "I just can't understand why Schrang don't want to work with me," he said.

"Because you are a piece of shit," said the good Lieutenant Marine. "Now get your fat blubbering ass out of here and back on the bus or I'll have you arrested for assaulting Schrang. Not that anyone in his or her right mind would believe that. But let's see your retired Supreme Court judge father help get you out of central booking."

I looked at Freddie, smiled, "Thanks, I could not have said it better." I walked out the door whistling. It was another beautiful star-filled night at Bellevue.

On our unit we had a goldfish named Zee. We kept it in a bowl in one of the upper cabinets between the dressings.

One night Fat Joe and I got a call for a stabbing. We pulled up to the scene and Fat Joe placed the patient in the back of our bus. The patient was indeed sliced and diced several times. The EMTs arrived and we were in the process of stripping him down, assessing him, putting him on oxygen, and getting a line into him. The guy was intoxicated and was somewhat combative.

I finally told the patient, "Hey, calm the fuck down and look at the fish."

"What the fuck you talkin' 'bout?"

"Up there. Look at the fish. This guy has shit for veins," I said, looking on both arms for access.

"Who you saying has shit for brains?" he asked indignantly.

"I didn't say *shit for brains*. I said, *shit for veins*. Just keep looking at the goldfish." He turned his neck and saw the fish in the bowl

"You're out of your . . . ow," he yelled, as I stuck a fourteen-gauge into his neck

"Why you do that?" he asked.

"Cause I care."

"You one crazy son of a bitch," he muttered, not giving us any more problems as he watched the fish swim merrily in its bowl.

A lieutenant ordered us to take the 10Z goldfish off. He had heard that ISU, also known as Becker's Gestapo, was on the prowl. We were ordered to keep the goldfish in the medic room where our drugs were stored. One day I came off a tour and saw the empty bowl. I asked the lieutenant where the fish was. He smiled and said he found it dead, so he flushed it down the toilet.

"Why didn't you start CPR?" I asked, as I walked out to the unit.

Simeon Klebner was a dispatcher at this time. When he heard what happened, he sent the following message citywide: "We regret the passing of the 10 Zebra goldfish. Services will be held with a rolling bar in the Bellevue Paramedic Restock Room after 01:00 hours." The crews loved it, but the gods and wannabe gods went berserk

It had been a long, not-too-eventful night in "Dominican Land," the upper West Side of Manhattan where we were deployed. I was driving and watching Fat Joe as he tried to impress the beautiful full-bodied

Dominican girls. Here the Latin beat, the rhythm of life itself, could be felt invigorating the hardworking community. But there was a dark side.

Earlier in the evening, while we were having coffee at the Dunkin' Donuts across from Columbia Presbyterian Medical Center at 168th Street and Broadway, we noticed New York's Finest and DEA agents pull over and search five cars at a time. They made some arrests. Ninety percent of the boys and girls in the cars were white and had New Jersey plates.

Our tour was nearly over as we started to re-deploy ourselves on the computer. A cold rain fell for a short while and then subsided. As I drove down Broadway we heard a "Shooting" assigned to a Basic unit from Harlem. We were four blocks out when Fat Joe asked if I wanted to take the job. I turned the bus around and started to accelerate, throwing on the lights and siren. Fat Joe put us on the job and notified the dispatcher. He was trying to show me how much of a real medic he could be.

"I hope a lot of people are shot!" he said excitedly. I didn't even look at him; I was just hoping the shooter would still be on the scene with one round left in the chamber, after asshole's last statement. We arrived and were the only unit there, so I got out to check what was happening.

"She's shot," screamed a male. "Hurry!"

The scene was pandemonium. People were running, pushing, and crying.

"There's more people shot upstairs," a kid told me as he ran out of the building. After realizing it was a walkup to the dance floor, Fat Joe made the command decision like a real *senior medic* of his caliber.

"I'll stay here with the shot girl."

I didn't answer him as I grabbed the trauma bag and headed up the two flights of stairs to the club, alone. I found myself as the only white in a sea of confused, scared black teens.

"Make way," one guy screamed.

"Let the paramedic in," another yelled as he attempted to push back the crowd.

"Over here! Over here, please," a girl called out. I moved toward the voice but was unable to see the girl. Stepping over turned chairs and tables, I walked on. After what seemed like years, two young men helped me to locate the girl who was calling out to me.

She was cradling the victim. He was a good-looking boy, about sixteen or seventeen. Judging from his build, he must have been into sports. His gray tuxedo jacket was pulled back with the red corsage still attached to the lapel. The white frilled shirt had two massive red blotches of blood in the upper chest area. His lifeless eyes looked unblinkingly, as tears from the girl holding him dripped onto his face. Blood mixed with brain matter was oozing from his mouth and was forming globs of bright red and gray staining her young hands and lavender dress.

I reached down and felt for a pulse. It was a show of compassion for her and to confirm what she already knew. In volatile situations like this, if I just walked away from the body without making an overt gesture of compassion, it could blow up and be directed toward me. The rescuer can become the victim

Her eyes were so young and filled with the terror of knowing. Pleading, our eyes met as I knelt down.

"I'm sorry, very sorry," I whispered, tenderly touching her shoulder. She collapsed into a bundle of crushed dreams, holding the lifeless body even closer. I looked at two kids standing in the crowd. "I've got to check on the others. Please help her." They nodded.

It has always amazed me how in all the chaos, pain, and destruction, paramedics and EMTs find unselfish people of courage who help us. The sad part is that we never get a chance to thank them

"Over here," said a young man. On the floor, about thirty feet from the first victim, lay another young man.

"Yo little brother, how are you doing?" I asked as I scanned his body. He had blood in the stomach area as well as his upper left chest area. The kid was extremely diaphoretic. One of the young men had been holding a package of cigarettes over the hole in his chest, actually buying the victim enough time for me to get there. This was preventing air from entering the boy's chest and collapsing his lung and crushing his heart. This condition is known as a pneumothorax. If it involves blood entering the lungs, it is a hemothorax. If both, as I suspected in this case, it would be a pneumo/hemothorax.

"Get me to the fuckin' hospital," the kid demanded. I ignored him since he was talking and had a good mental status. This told me he had at least an eighty-palp blood pressure and I still had time to work on him. I looked up and saw the banner and balloons. It was their prom night with one dead so far.

"Hey guys, I'll need some help," I said. "You keep holding those cigarettes there until I get him stripped. Ever think of becoming a doctor? You did a great job," I said as I cut the kid's shirt from his body, revealing an evisceration, a rupture of the abdominal wall that allows the abdominal contents to escape through the hole.

"No, I'm into computers but my dad was a medic in Nam. He worries about me so he taught me first aid since I was a kid. How's it looking?"

"Interesting. That's part of his bowel, protruding out. We have work to do."

With the shirt cut away, I applied an occlusive dressing over the hole in his chest. The kid wasn't having any problems with his lungs since he kept mouthing off.

"Yo, yo, mother fucker. Stop playing doctor. Get me to the fuckin' hospital now!"

"Guys, we are going to have to roll him to the right. I need you to hold his head, and you his hips. On three we roll him and keep him straight. I have to see where these bullets went, okay?" The kids nodded.

"Yo, ambulance driver. Get me to the hospital, you, mother fucker."

"Yo, Bean. The medic is trying to help you. Chill," one kid said impatiently.

"One, two, three, roll him. Good, hold him there. I found the exit for one round." One had exited his right scapular area, and I knew it had done neurological damage by the way his right arm was limp. After patching the wound, we rolled him back and I prepared to place two IVs.

"Yo, Whitie. Get me." He didn't continue.

"Shut up, nigger! The man and all of us are working to save your life."

"You ain't puttin' that in me, mother fucker."

"Okay, that's it. You want to die?" I didn't give him time to answer. "Shut the fuck up or I'll gag you. Understand?" I dropped two fourteen-gauge large catheters into him, giving me IV access. Then I checked his blood pressure and lungs again.

"He's over there," I heard someone yell. Much to my delight, the cavalry was there to save the day.

Two Harlem EMTs approached with two cops. The EMTs never let us paramedics forget that: Paramedics save the patients, but the EMTs save the paramedics. God bless their little Piss Patch Souls.

The EMTs gently loaded him onto the long board and collared him to keep spinal stabilization.

"Where we going, Jim?" asked the EMT.

"Harlem."

All of a sudden, this loudmouth kid starts crying, "No! Please, not Harlem. I don't want to go."

"Hold up," I said. "Not Harlem, huh?"

"No, please, Saint Luke's."

I directed the crew to lower him back to the floor. The crew and the two cops were really concerned about this move, but there was a lesson this lad needed to learn.

"Okay, Mr. Hot Shot. You realize you'll die if we take you to Harlem, right?"

"Yes," he answered, bawling like a baby.

"Okay. We will take you to Saint Luke's only after you apologize to me in front of your friends and thank them for helping you. It's either that or this white mother fuckin' ambulance driver will take your black ass to Harlem where you'll . . . die. Now let's hear it? I'm sorry, Mr. White motherfuckin' Paramedic."

The kid started, "I'm sorry Mr. White motherfuckin' Paramedic. Please take me to Saint Luke's, I want to live."

"And what about these young gentlemen?"

"I'm sorry. Thank you for helping me."

"All right. The nigger thanked us home boys for helping save his life," one of the kids said.

"Okay, let's get the gentleman to Harlem," I said, as I looked at his eyes becoming big and round. Before he could say anything, I bent over, looked into his eyes and said with a smile, "I mean Saint Luke's." He smiled and reached for my hand with his functional left hand.

We headed on downstairs and into the back of the BLS unit. When the EMT crew had first arrived, one of them had asked Fat Joe where I was.

He told them, "Up there, with some people shot." The EMT looked at Fat Joe's shot female. All it required was a band-aid. I looked over at him, sitting like King Tub on a milk crate, talking to the girl. I wiped the sweat from my weary eyes and closed the doors as we drove off. Fat Joe, on seeing the unit leave, got right on the radio demanding more units and a supervisor.

"My partner has left me here alone with a shot female!" I heard him say as I turned off the radio.

A Basic unit from Bellevue brought a tight asthmatic into Beekman Hospital in lower Manhattan. As usual, the staff ignored the crew and the patient. Finally, an EMT got on his radio and called for a medic unit forthwith. He stated he was in the emergency room, the staff was inattentive, and his patient was about to code. One Oh Zee came on the air and responded. Izzi Huckster was one of the medics. As they turned the corner in the small ER, the two medics saw the frantic concern on the EMTs' faces as the patient coded

Now the staff wanted to play. One EMT jumped up and pushed the staff away, as his partner helped the medics with the patient in respiratory arrest on the floor. As the doctors and nurses ran for security, the EMT called for a supervisor. The boss, a very rare one in EMS Land, responded. When he got there, two EMTs were getting physical with the staff and security, who were interfering with the medic's ability providing patient care. The lieutenant from the downtown station told the staff and security to back off or he would call the police.

The doctors yelled that the patient was theirs and should be surrendered. Lieutenant Juan "Tony" Torres from Station Eleven asked the medics what they wanted to do. In unison they said they were *taking the patient to Bellevue*. And indeed they did. Beekman was closed by the State, while an investigation was conducted. Beekman reopened after being fined.

These were the respected crews of Stress Free. These were men who made decisions and went to the wall for the patients. As for Tony, well, he was a rare breed on this job.

As an intro into the next story, I must first tell you a story that happened many years ago when I was a County Mountie. We were called to aid a "Sick Child." As we entered the well-kept apartment, a police officer was consoling a chunky, forty-year-old female who was crying hysterically.

Upon seeing us, she cried, "He raped her! He raped her."

"Where's the victim?" my partner asked.

"It's the kid," the officer said in a matter-of-fact tone.

My partner stayed with the hysterical woman. The ten-year-old, who stood about four and a half feet tall, was standing by another officer. She had rich, midnight black skin with braided hair beautifully decorated with colorfully vibrant beads. Dark brown eyes were dramatically offset by the white sclera sunken in a round face with pudgy cheeks.

She stood quietly while I knelt down, introduced myself, and asked if she was hurt or bleeding? "Yes" was the reply in an angelic voice. Explaining my concern, I asked if it would be okay if I checked her. The child softly whispered "yes," reaching for my hand, so we proceeded into the bedroom with another officer. Again I explained what I had to do and that I'd need her help. She nodded.

As she lay on the bed, I gently examined her, placing a dressing on a still bleeding vagina. While working, I asked questions in a low, soothing voice. The cop was taking notes as she explained that she had seen the man by her school. When she came home he knocked, asking for a drink of water. The child, realizing how hot the day had been, let him in, getting a glass of cold water. After the drink, he struck. As I continued to ask, the cop nodded his approval. Establishing the location of the assault as the bedroom, I noticed a jar on the counter. The little girl explained the perpetrator had used Vaseline on his penis before entering her. I looked at the cop who nodded and smiled. Both of us knew the jar of Vaseline had the perpetrator's fingerprints on it.

"Nice going," he said, as I dressed her.

The girl was most concerned her friends would find out about the incident while she was being carried to the ambulance. As we took her to the bus, residents and friends in the lobby asked exactly that. I told them she was sick. In the bus, I received a big smile and a kiss from the little treasure. Several weeks later, the perpetrator was captured, thanks to the fingerprints and the little girl's power of observation to look deeper.

On the whole, the public never was dull. We met people from all walks of life and not at their best. There were cases that hurt because of the senseless trauma caused by egotistical hatred. Unless you work in a small, low-call-volume area, I think you will agree that there are jobs you would like to follow up on, but just never get to. It was during my tour on 10Z that I started to formulate the idea of making a book. Cops, as well as EMS working the ghetto, not only observed the raw, extreme depravity of human experience, but, if honest to self, realized we were no less a part of it than the individuals we served. Unlike the aforementioned case early in my career in which the "bad guy" was caught, in the following story who really is the "bad guy"? Look deeper, much deeper, because nothing is ever as it appears. Thus, over the years, I interviewed the patients, victims, families, friends, perps and cops of some of the most microbic cases. Below is one such story, but really nothing new for ghetto medics, EMTs and cops.

She hurried home from school, petting the family dog, Cookie. Then, ditching her books, she grabbed a sip of ice tea from the refrigerator, gave Cookie some water, and ran to the bathroom. Checking herself out for a big date with Raymond, she changed her blouse, stopping to look at her slim form in the mirror. She stood about five feet three inches, with a brown silky complexion, her dark eyes sparkling above a beautiful smile that exposed glittering white teeth. She borrowed some of her mother's perfume, lipstick, and eyeliner, which was forbidden.

Her mother was working late at the hospital and would not be home for several hours. She knew her mother would call about 10:00 P.M.., but she would be home way before then. Her older brother, Charlie, was working at the store and would be in by eight. He was such a pain, she thought to herself. He had actually hit her several times, claiming that she was too young to hang out. She had learned long ago not to fight Charlie, but to listen to him. If need be, submit to his punishing, no matter what he did. She knew he loved her and kept his word about not telling her mother when she got into trouble at school.

But tonight was her night. There was no school tomorrow. She would be able to spend time with Raymond. She'd had a crush on him since school started several months ago. Charlie hadn't found out about Raymond yet. If he found out that a seventeen-year-old homeboy liked his thirteen-year-old kid sister, Charlie would've killed him. It did not matter about the age. It was because Charlie hated drug dealers and drunks.

At sixteen, Charlie still silently pondered his father coming home drunk or high, smoking weed, and beating his mother if she didn't "perform." At the tender age of eight, Charlie remembered being knocked unconscious after a futile attempt to defend her, but not before being stripped and raped in front of both mother and sister. He recalled the fear of waking up in the back of an ambulance as a paramedic placed an IV in his arm. His mother begged him not to say anything since she knew the family would be separated, and finally retaliation would be death for all of them. Thus nothing came of the case. Charlie, as well as the mother, silently submitted to the father's escalating sexual and violent, demonic rage. He watched his father's mind sink deeper into depravity until, one fateful night, his father took a knife, threatening both mother and sister. Tomica lay huddled in a fetal position on the couch, crying. Their mother having been knocked to the floor, realizing his intent, lunged onto the couch to protect the terrified child.

Charlie ran to the kitchen, grabbing a meat cleaver. As his father raised the knife above his head, Charlie violently drove the cleaver into his father's back as deep as it would go. The man dropped the knife. As the father turned slowly, Charlie no longer recognized the glazed eyes of the man trying to reach behind his back to get the cleaver. The gaunt, diaphoretic face suddenly took on a terrified expression. A final gasp came from his blood-tinged dry lips before crashing to the floor, dead.

Tomica looked up from her mother's breast to see the red blotch grow into a larger pool swallowing their father. Charlie stood stoic, staring. He was eleven years old and his sister was nine.

Things had been better since that day a lifetime ago. Charlie became the man of the house, working odd jobs while continuing to attend school. If Tomica was late, got involved in a fight, or back-talked their mother, Charlie would punish her. The young girl accepted this and blossomed; life was indeed good.

Tomica was gifted in writing and hoped one day to write romance novels. She had several articles published in the school's newspaper. Today Tawanna, one of Raymond's old girlfriends, had threatened her outside of English class.

Tawanna said that Raymond wanted to meet Tomica by the river at 4:00 P.M. She warned Tomica not to go. Tomica knew the place well and blew off the threat, promising, "No one will keep me from *my* Raymond."

Tomica ran to her mother's room, put on her mom's favorite gold earrings, and dashed out the door. It would take some time to get to the river location in the Park by the Third Avenue Bridge. Tomica enjoyed each step as she walked in the crisp fall air. Life was so promising, so good.

As Tomica drew close to the specified location, she was approached by Sandra, another thirteen-year-old, who told her she would accompany her to Raymond. She followed Sandra under the bridge. At the base of the bridge was a large room used to store equipment for bridge maintenance.

"Go right in," Sandra said. Something didn't seem right.

"I'll wait out here for Raymond, thanks," Tomica said, starting to turn to look at the gray blue water.

"Oh no, you won't, bitch," Tawanna said, as she stepped from the shadows. Tomica's heart raced, realizing the trap had been sprung. She spun on her heels and started to run. She was only able to take two steps before Sandra punched her in the face with a closed fist, stunning her. At the same moment, Tawanna grabbed her from behind, pulling her into the room. Tomica attempted to break free by wiggling out of her coat.

Tawanna screamed, "Get the bitch. She's getting away."

All at once, it seemed like there were numerous hands grabbing her as she attempted to fight and scream. A cloth bag was dropped over her head and a hand covered her mouth. She was being suffocated, and she stopped resisting.

"Got her," came the victory yell from Tawanna, as she pulled Tomica backward into the large, dank room. Once they were inside, the steel door crashed shut, sending a chill through Tomica, as if her fate had been sealed. She stood erect. No hands held her now. After several agonizing minutes of silence, she reached up to remove the hood. She was struck in the stomach and her petite body crashed to the concrete floor.

"So you want to see what's going on? Stand up, Tomica," was the command. "Remove the bag," Tawanna ordered. It was pulled off and it took a minute for Tomica's eyes to adjust to the harsh light from the naked bulbs hanging from the wires that crisscrossed the ceiling. As she focused, the stark light cast shadows, mimicking her grim situation.

"I told you to stay away from my man, bitch. Didn't I?" demanded Tawanna.

Realizing she was out of her league, Tomica looked at the ten girls who made up the family and she started to cry.

"Yes," she said in a wavering voice.

Smash, right across the face came the smack from Tawanna. As Tomica's head spun, Sandra yanked her hair from behind.

"No tears when speaking to the lady, understand?"

"Yes," came an even weaker-sounding answer.

"You are being tried by my family for offenses against them," Tawanna bellowed.

"But . . . ," Tomica doubled up from the shot to her stomach. Hands pulled her to her feet as her head was pulled upright.

"I don't have no time for you, bitch. Hey, the little bitch be wearing eyeliner and smells like a real ho."

Tomica's eyeliner ran down her face as she fought back the tears. Tawanna, a far heavier girl and two inches taller, stood in front of her as the girls held Tomica's arms at her side.

"You going to do my man?" she asked softly.

"No," came Tomica's honest answer. She was still a virgin at thirteen.

"So you don't think my man is good enough for you, do you, ho? Is that what you say?" demanded Tawanna.

"Wow, she dissin' you sister," someone said.

"No . . . I didn't mean . . ." Before she could say another word, a knife was at her throat and she froze. Tawanna toyed with the petrified girl, moving the blade up and down her neck. "Please, plea . . ."

"The bitch is beggin'," they laughed. "Now I'm a lady, the man's lady. That means I'm fair, right?"

"Right lady," the family chimed in.

"I'm going to give you a chance, ho. Am I good to you or not?" she asked Tomica, her black eyes flashing in an uncontrollable rage. The knife at Tomica's throat caused her neck to arch back. "Now, you are going to do as I say. Everything, right?" she asked, with a grin on her face, turning to her crew.

"I'll do whatever you want," Tomica said.

"Good, because tonight you will be my ho. Now, Jenny, you start the video going." Jenny got the camera out as the girls started laughing and a large black Rotweiller started growling and barking from the corner.

"Hush up, Blackie," Tawanna commanded, as she walked over and smacked the large dog on the snout.

Jenny got the camera ready and Tawanna returned to stand in front of Tomica and said, "Give the bitch room. She is happy. I'm giving her a break." Once Jenny was ready and the family had stepped back, Tawanna stood next to Jenny.

"You shooting?"

"Yeah."

"Okay ho, say your name."

"Tomica White," she said meekly, as her eyes darted around the room.

"Okay, Miss Ho White, take your clothes off for my man. Give him a good show." As Tomica froze, it all became clear. Raymond was never interested in her. He just wanted Tawanna to enjoy herself, and Tawanna was going to give him a gift, the video of her.

"I . . . I . . . can't."

"Okay, stop taping. The ho needs some motivation."

As Tawanna approached, Tomica felt a chill run down her spine and she attempted to step back.

"Hold her." Several girls grabbed Tomica as Tawanna brought the knife to her throat. "Here's your motivation, bitch." In one lightning flash, she moved the knife up slicing Tomica's right cheek. Blood ran down Tomica's swan-like neck. The slice was about two inches long and was superficial, but Tomica froze. Tawanna grabbed the frightened girl by the hair. As the blood ran down her check, she felt it form a pool on her neck. Her lacy, white blouse absorbed the blood like a bib. Terrified beyond words, Tomica stood frozen, unable to move. Her legs felt weak, her throat instantly dry, and she could hardly breathe.

"Now I'm a lady, The Man's lady," Tawanna said in a shy, toying manner, smiling to her family. She violently yanked Tomica's head harder.

"Now since I'm a lady. The man's lady, you're going to do as I say."

She licked the wound with her thick tongue. The blood now covered her mouth and chin. Tawanna looked into the girl's frightened eyes.

"Kiss me," she ordered. The petrified girl complied. Still holding her, she said, "And now that you have insulted me again, you will do as you are told. Correct?" she bellowed.

"Yes," came the whisper as her neck muscles burned and spasmed from the position she was in. There was silence in the room.

"Okay, strip." Slowly Tomica started to remove her blouse. Once it was off, with the camera going, Tawanna said, "And the pants for my man." Tomica slowly opened her skintight jeans and slid them down to her ankles and stood up.

"Tomica, what's your best subject?"

"English," she responded, looking awkward and lost. Tawanna walked around the girl examining her as she stood there in her bra and panties, jeans at her feet covering the new white sneakers Charles had bought her.

"Well, ho, if you understand English, and that's your best subject, what the fuck are your ass-hugging jeans still doing on?" With this, Tawanna, who was behind her, smacked her in the back of the head, sending her crashing to the floor.

"I said, get them off!"

As Tomica attempted to rapidly pull them off, Tawanna said, "Give the bitch a hand." Several girls rushed forward in a frenzy. They pushed her onto her back as they pulled her jeans and sneakers off.

"Hey, these will fit," shouted one girl, as they split up her jeans and sneakers.

"Stand up for the lady," screamed Sandra, who received a smile from Tawanna. Once on her feet, Tomica looked down at the floor, hands to her side now, wishing she had listened to Charlie or that somehow, someway, he would find her. The floor felt cool even with her socks on, though her body felt like it was burning from the assaults.

"Okay, Miss Ho White, or is that Snow White?" Tawanna said as they all laughed. Without looking up she undid her bra and dropped it to the floor.

"Wait. Wait," yelled Sandra, who appeared to be second in charge. "You're stripping for 'The Man.' 'The Lady's Man.' Look up," she said, as she reached across and squeezed her facial cheeks.

"This girl is really dissin' The Lady," one girl said. Tomica just stood there.

"Ladies, my family. I thank you for being hurt by my hurt. But I'm The Lady, The Man's Lady, and this bitch will pay. But first let's play."

She looked at the dazed girl who stood in front of her. Even with her running eyeliner and blood on her mouth, the gracefulness was still there. Her body was beautifully sculptured. Her breasts were firm and small. White lace panties set off her skin. Even her socks with the pompoms set off long, slender, chocolate legs. Tawanna hated everything about Tomica. She was smart and beautiful.

"Okay, Tomica." This was the first time she called her by her name. "Look at the camera and get those fuckin' white panties off."

Tomica's eyes burned with rage as she defiantly pulled her panties off. This slight act of anger was not missed.

"Turn for the camera, bitch."

Tomica complied, with her slender fingers interwoven and covering her love mound below her flat stomach. Tawanna walked up and signaled with her head. Several girls approached, grabbing Tomica.

"Think you're special? You gonna do my man?" Tawanna asked coyly.

Tomica did not answer.

"You better answer The Lady, The Man's Lady, bitch," said a girl. Tomica stood there.

"So you were going to do him, huh?"

"No, I was not. Nor would I. You can have him, you sick bitch," Tomica yelled in a sudden rage of defiance.

"Bitch? I can have him. You think you're too good for him, don't you, Tomica ho White?" Tawanna screamed, flying into a rage, twisting her head and facial muscles as she got within one inch of the defiant Tomica. The camera rolled.

"Well, since you are so graciously giving me the man, I'll give you someone special, Blackie," she screamed as the dog barked and pulled on its chain.

Reality thundered across Tomica's brain. "Oh God. Not the dog. Plea—" Tawanna grabbed her face and squeezed it so hard she couldn't finish her sentence.

"So you wouldn't do The Man?"

"Please I'll do . . ." She froze in mid-sentence as she looked into Tawanna's cold calculating eyes.

"Kiss me, ho," she said, as the family applauded. "I want your lips parted."

"Which ones?" one girl yelled as everyone laughed.

"Hold her," Tawanna said, as she started to kiss Tomica, forcibly opening her lips with her tongue before rapidly ending the kiss. "The ho likes this. Again!"

This time there was little resistance as Tawanna's tongue entered Tomica's mouth, playing with her tongue. At the same time she reached down and attempted to finger the girl's love mound. Tomica attempted to voice a protest and close her legs. The family had other ideas. Tawanna opened her eyes long enough to look over at Sandra and then into the open eyes of the squirming Tomica. The family had spread the girl's legs apart and Tawanna was beginning to gently massage the outer lips.

Tawanna broke the kiss long enough to look down at her fingers then said, "Again," as Tomica's head was pulled back. Tawanna entered the girl's mouth, finding less resistance. Two of the family had reached over and were massaging and nibbling at her breasts. As Tawanna worked her tongue, her finger was now at work entering the parting lips of the girl's love mound and found its mark. Slowly, in a rhythmic pattern to match her tongue's movement, she massaged the clit. Tomica's body was now betraying her will as she became moist and was violated deeper.

Tawanna would never admit it, but she enjoyed everything about this moment with Tomica. Tomica's tongue was now starting to move as well as her hips swaying. She was lost in this unknown, captivating energy. It built up until, in one split second, her legs gave way as she arched backward in her first orgasm coming down hard on Tawanna's finger. Tomica attempted to arch again as Tawanna's finger violently penetrated her vagina, breaking her hymen.

The girl was still held by the family. Tawanna, her finger still in place, commanded, "Again." After two more robust orgasms, they dropped Tomica to the floor. As they stepped away from her, she curled into the fetal position.

Tomica didn't hear the call for the ropes. She didn't even realize the family was moving around until she felt them grab her arms and start dragging her.

"What? What are you doing?" she asked, in a startled voice. No one answered. There was no strength in her, as she looked over her shoulder and saw her final destination, four u-bolts in the floor. The family spread her arms and legs, tying them with the rope to the bolts.

"She might pull out of the ropes. Use the cuffs," one girl said. As she lay on the floor, she watched as each hand was handcuffed to a bolt in the concrete floor. She attempted to pull free, but it was a futile gesture.

"We still good on the film?" asked Sandra.

"Yeah, we have plenty."

Tawanna walked over, stopped, and looked at the young girl. Without a sound, she took out her knife as she knelt down beside her. There was a deafening silence as Tawanna slowly, methodically ran the side of the knife across the terrified girl's nose down across her lips, parting them and moving next to her throat. Tomica dared not swallow. The girl's respirations increased, her breasts rising up with each breath.

As the knife meandered down her body, Tomica turned to Tawanna. The cold knife raised her nipples and Tawanna stopped and looked into her eyes. At that moment, she looked back to her knife as it trailed across the girl's flat stomach to her love mound. Tawanna knelt there, covered in sweat as her fear rose.

Tawanna, a master of fear, slid the side of the knife along the moistened, bloodied outer lips of the girl's vagina. Tomica initially attempted to withdraw, but couldn't because of the restraints to her outstretched legs. Tawanna brought the moistened knife up and examined it. She saw the bloodied fluid on it. She said to Tomica in a soft, almost sorrowful voice, "Lick it clean."

Tomica complied.

"Let me see your tongue. All the way out." Tomica complied. "Good." She placed the knife on Tomica's flat stomach, bent over, and kissed her. Tawanna's tongue searched and found Tomica's tongue, enjoying the succulent juices. Next, she tenderly kissed the girl's ears and neck and then moved to her breasts. One of the girls started to say something and Tawanna shot her a look. "Just keep the camera going," she said in a soft seductive voice.

As she worked on the outstretched body of the girl, Tomica started to physically respond with a moan and whimper. Lower Tawanna went, working, and caressing the straining girl. Tawanna stopped and looked at Tomica, whose head turned to the side as she released another moan. Their eyes met. Tawanna tenderly moved the younger, smaller girl's black hair from her face. For what seemed like an eternity both looked. Tawanna delving into Tomica's soul, seeing it filled with fear, but surrendering to the onslaught of passion.

Tomica was trying desperately to please, but was confused at enjoying her captor's games of passion. She searched Tawanna's eyes for a glimmer of hope, but saw only sorrow, regret. As their eyes were locked, Tawanna worked gently on Tomica's thighs and now her honey pot with her right hand. Tomica responded. Tawanna positioned herself and kissed the girl's navel, running her tongue slowly along her hip, sending a shudder through the girl. Tawanna nibbled at the girl's feet and toes through her socks, eliciting a childlike giggle from her prisoner. Tomica raised her head. An ever so slight smile crossed her lips as Tawanna worked toward her sweet honey pot. When the girl's virginal lips were touched by her captor's darting tongue, it sent electrifying bolts up the unsuspecting Tomica's spine. Her body shook uncontrollably from the breathtaking spasms rocketing her head back, crashing against the floor.

Tomica was lost in an ecstasy. She rocked violently against the restraints, thrashing her head from side to side in repeated uncontrolled spasms of pleasure. Tawanna sensed her control over her prisoner, as she quickly looked up, and then returned to the job at hand. It was a combination hand and tongue job. Tawanna's tongue worked the girl's lips and clit like a master craftsman. She moistened her fingers in some of the girl's hot love juices exploding in an eternal gushing stream from her love fountain. When her fingers were moistened, she increased her tongue action to a fever pitch. When she sensed Tomica could stand no more she forcibly entered her rectum and vagina simultaneously. Tomica let out a loud moan. The onslaught continued at lightning speed with Tomica trying to catch her breath. As suddenly as lightning was gone, Tawanna stopped. Tomica fought to catch her breath and get her brain grounded again. Tawanna stood above her.

Before she could say anything, Tawanna snapped her fingers and Blackie barked. Tomica attempted to blow her hair out of her face, when she felt the dog lick her leg.

"I'll help you with the hair, ho," said Sandra, as she brushed the girl's hair back. "We want you nice and pretty for this."

Tomica rapidly turned her head and screamed, "Tawanna, Please. I'm begging. No," she cried as their eyes met.

"Listen," Tawanna started in a sad voice, "I'm The Lady. 'The Lady of the Man'. Now you were good, better than most. But you dissed me, and my family. My family, we are all we have, girl." There was a thoughtful pause. She walked over, reached down, took the girl's socks off. "Open your mouth." Tomica did, as the tears rolled down her cheeks. Tawanna put the socks in the girl's mouth. "If you're a good lay and Blackie don't rip the socks out of your mouth, it will be over after he has his fun. If he don't feel you've been good to him . . . well, if he gets these socks from your mouth you'll need to service him more." She stood up.

Tomica looked up at the ceiling then screamed through the gags as the gigantic dog lurched forward, sniffing and licking her moist honey pot. She thrashed wildly, her neck veins bulging as her head shot up. At this point Blackie was pulled away. Thinking she had received a reprieve, Tomica started to cry. Several family members pulled up a large car seat they were sitting on and flipped it over. They pulled up the girl, bent her over and tied her. With her legs tied apart, her butt in the air, she knew what was about to happen. Her eyes expanded grotesquely from their sockets as the dog mounted her, to the roar of the family. He had no problem in finding his mark and she screamed in agony, as it felt like he was ripping her apart.

To get better leverage the gigantic beast placed two large paws on her shoulders. When they slipped off her wet, thrashing body he demonically repositioned them on the girl's back. Turning her head, she looked over her shoulder into the dog's eyes. As Tomica's eyes met his, she knew she was gazing into hell. The dog continued his icy stare into her soul as he pounded her. She was transfixed with paralyzing fear. She lay on her stomach unable to breathe from the weight of the mammoth paws and nails digging into her back. The dog's warm drool slid down her face. Tomica did not move. She could not break the stare of this dog from hell.

“Okay, enough for the fun, roll her over,” Tawanna said.

Tomica was oblivious and didn’t feel the girls as they rolled her onto her stomach, replacing the handcuffs. Sandra was the first to approach and produce her friend, a razor blade. Tomica just lay there as Sandra sliced ever so lightly into the girl’s back drawing blood. Yes the blood feast had begun. Each girl had her turn. When they were finished they turned her over. There was no resistance as they signed for the family. Then they looked at their work. They had passed judgment. On the cold, blood-stained floor lay an unresponsive, naked thirteen-year-old girl. Every square inch of her body had the family signature, including the soles of her feet and face. Blood ran from her ear lobes where her mother’s gold earrings had been “sliced” free.

“Okay, let’s get out of here, family business is adjourned,” Tawanna said.

“Are we going to leave her here?” asked a girl.

“No, stupid,” said Sandra, “we’ll let her swim like that crying bitch Rhonda last summer.”

“Oh, yeah.”

They lifted her up, untying her feet and undoing the cuffs.

“Do you want the cuffs back on?”

“No, I don’t want to lose another set on a bitch. Just tie her hands,” Tawanna ordered, as she walked over and opened the door. It was dark now and colder. Some homeless people wandered around.

“Put her coat around her and let’s get her to the river now. I don’t want no one spying us,” she commanded. Several girls lifted Tomica to the standing position. They tied rope around her hands in the front of her. Next, they draped her coat over her sliced shoulders and walked her to the churning East River. They laughed as they pushed the compliant Tomica off the eight-foot embankment. There was a splash as they saw her coat float up to the surface.

At that moment they heard sirens. All the girls screamed and began running in all directions, like roaches. They soon realized the cops were on a run, speeding across the bridge overhead, and not after them.

"Let's get some chicken," someone suggested as they walked away.

When Tomica hit the water, a kaleidoscope of energies erupted. Her body screamed from the pain of the salt water entering the signatures all over her mutilated body. She gasped for air, receiving cold, oily water instead. With some unknown help, she felt her body being caressed as it was moving sideways and upward. Her feet were now kicking to keep the momentum going. She could feel as the current acted like magic fingers, untying the rope binding her wrist. Suddenly, like a Polaris missile launched from a submarine, she shot up, breaking the surface of the turbulent river, gasping for air. The night was dark, but she saw lights as she grabbed onto the piling she was hurled against. Again, an unseen force helped push her out of the river. She was naked and freezing. She stumbled toward some lights, leaving a bloody trail from her feet on the fresh dusting of snow covering the concrete.

The bus driver almost hit her as he pulled his bus from the terminal. He took off his jacket and walked the speechless girl into the office.

Stress Free responded to the scene. The crew was no longer amazed at the depravity in human suffering. The girl wouldn't talk, but followed commands. She was taken to Harlem Hospital where she was identified and her mother and brother were called.

Days passed, but she only stared at the ceiling. Charlie placed fresh flowers next to her bed and talked to her, as he held her hand. One day he walked in and said the name Tawanna and Tomica's eyes flashed. Charlie looked around, then back at his sister. Slowly he reached up and pulled down the white sheet covering her body. He had done this before, as if burning the image of her sliced body into his mind. But this time, after getting the response concerning Tawanna, he looked at her exposed chest and saw different marks, other than the slices.

"Blackie," he whispered. Tomica's eyes flashed again in terror, then returned to staring at the ceiling. She heard Charlie crying and felt his warm tears splash on her naked chest as he held her. Gently he covered her and then kissed her.

"I'll get them, all of them," he said as he walked from the room for the last time.

As she lay there she thought Charlie will be going to jail for murder, and it's my fault. For the first time in several days she couldn't focus on the chipped white ceiling above her as tears rolled down her swollen, scarred cheeks.

Sometimes helpers come in all shapes and sizes. Paramedic Oz was a very special paramedic. He got his name from working with me on Stress Free 10Z. He was a hand puppet, stethoscope and all.

One day Paramedic Oz was on patrol with my partner and me in Manhattan, when we got a call for a "Pedestrian Struck." My partner Jack put away his freshly purchased Chinese dinner as we pulled up to the Basic unit. The Bellevue EMTs had done a good job of evaluating the patient. However, the patient, a black male, was not cooperating and just lay there.

He was a cab driver who got into a confrontation with a motorist. Being new to America and having watched all those movies we send abroad, the driver climbed out of his cab to do battle, just like in the movies. Suddenly the vehicle took off, our new immigrant American, who wanted to be a hero, threw himself onto the front of the moving vehicle just the way he witnessed heroes do in the movies. The vehicle accelerated down the street when it suddenly dawned on our hapless hero that movies are movies and this was real life. With that reality check our wannabee hero screamed hysterically for the driver to stop!

Well, this being New York, the driver did as requested and stopped. Unfortunately, our fearless cab driver didn't, until the asphalt of 5th. Avenue met him. The vehicle drove off. Gee, and they say NYC drivers don't follow directions!

The guy had a few bumps and bruises and was not cooperating. Was this secondary to some type of internal bleeding in the head or a crushing assault of the reality of the American film industry? On top of this, we were racing against a clock, to get Jack to his dinner before it grew cold. We do have priorities.

My partner, who was Little Buddha incarnate with untold patience, was starting to lose it. I said I'd get someone who could help us. A few moments later I returned. I told the cab driver to knock off the crap as I knelt on the floor on the side of the stretcher.

"If you refuse to talk to me, I will have no recourse. Paramedic Oz, who is getting pissed, will start an IV in your neck." With this, Paramedic Oz jumped onto this guy's chest and scared the hell out of him. The patient let out a hair-raising scream. His eyes became as wide as white dinner plates, trashing against the restraints, as he broke into a cold sweat, trying to get away from Paramedic Oz. Oh, he was now crying, but speaking the best English I'd ever heard. We left the patient in the care of the EMTs. Jack had his hot "Chinese" meal. What? Would you expect less from the Little Buddha?

In NYC EMS management there were assholes, then super assholes who tried their hardest to be at the top of the class. They didn't just screw up, they screwed up royally.

In 1988–1989, EMS decided to copy other systems and place two paramedics in a Jimmy type vehicle and call it a PRU (Paramedic Response Unit). The idea would have been great if it had been implemented correctly. The concept was to take paramedics out of an ambulance and place them in smaller vehicles. Thus if the job did not require paramedics, the patients would be turned over to the EMTs and transported to the hospital by them.

But leave it to the EMS chiefs to ruin anything that stands a chance of working. The vehicles could not transport anyone sick or injured. Thus we needed a Basic unit to respond with us on each call. Dual dispatching was the key. If the call was nonsense, you could pass it on to the Basic and be available to do what you were trained for, ALS (Advanced Life Support).

The idea was doomed from the start. Dispatchers would not always dispatch a dual response. With stellar dispatcher Mickey gone, so was good dispatching for the most part.

A typical EMS dispatcher was concerned with two things: clearing the board of jobs, not caring whether ALS or BLS gets assigned, and where's the food? This is not to say we didn't have some good dispatchers. But they were few and far between.

On top of this, the chief's own little battles spilled over. If the Chief of Operations wanted the PRU to work, he had to depend on the Chief of Communications working with him, which did not happen. Once again the gods of EMS fought, resulting in damage to paramedics and patient care. The PRU concept was great for the medics, a breath of fresh air.

Burnout was caused by continuously going to bullshit calls. A good example of this was the call type "Unconscious" and, adding salt to the wound, "It's an intox."

Under PRU, paramedics came to work more often and morale was better. Since medics got special incentives like the PRU, the EMTs wanted to stay on the job and become paramedics. Up to that point, anyone with three or four years on the job was considered strange. Most people left in fewer than three years.

To reiterate those proverbial words of paramedic Harvey Feintuck, "No good deed will go unpunished."

As the call volume increased, the PRU had to be replaced with a Basic unit, to reiterate, if it was to work. But, needless to say, the pundits never added the extra units. If it raised morale, gave incentives to EMS personnel, and provided better patient care, then it had to go.

With all the losers we had to contend with, we still kept our focus on patient care and humor.

One night, paramedic Nicola Halsey and I were with Lieutenant Rancier of Metropolitan Station Fifteen. Over the past few days, we had done more ALS than in a two-month period with an ambulance. As we stood talking to Lieutenant Rancier, he received a call that a Basic unit had a patient who needed to get to the hospital, but the patient had other ideas. Nor would he talk to our doctors in telemetry via phone. The good lieutenant asked us to take a ride with him, since he was an EMT and hoped we, as paramedics, could convince the patient to go, or at least talk to the doctor.

We grabbed our equipment and trudged up the stairs of a Harlem tenement. The hall was poorly lit when we reached the apartment. Standing to the side of the door, the lieutenant knocked with his flashlight.

The dilapidated door swung open and to our left we saw a black gentleman in his thirties sitting on a bed. The old, sheetless mattress had seen better days, as had he. Physically, this well-built guy could have played for the New York Jets. There were two EMTs, the gentleman's wife, and twelve-year-old stepdaughter in the room. The two EMTs explained the situation.

The patient was walking into the lobby when he got a glimpse of three neighborhood men, who struck him in the head with a heavy board and robbed him. When he came to, he found the broken board lying beside him. He struggled up the four flights to the apartment, where his wife wanted to call 911. He was adamant that she not call. As the man started to throw up and a black bump formed behind his ears, the wife called 911. His main concerns were losing his paycheck and getting revenge.

The lieutenant asked if the police had been called, but the look he received told the whole story. The quality of officers had changed through the years and not for the better. The cops were only interested in making overtime with a real collar, like a gun bust. The gentleman sat there and refused Lieutenant Rancier's attempts to convince him to talk to the doctor.

Nickie, my partner, decided to give it a shot since we both realized the man was critically injured. He had all the signs of a basilar skull fracture that would require surgery.

Nickie stood about five feet five inches, had shoulder-length blond hair, a beautiful tight body, and flashing blue eyes. A fiery English accent rolled off her tongue. She was a ravishing beauty with an attitude. This gorgeous paramedic kneeled down beside the patient, giving it all her charm and knowledge.

The guy wouldn't budge. "I'm not talken to no doctor, I'm not goin' to no hospital."

Never tell Nickie she couldn't do something. This was one case where she realized her limitation, blue eyes, blond hair, and all.

"Okay, there's only one thing left," I said, getting kind of tired of watching this guy fray off the good intentions of those who loved him. As Nickie got up, I placed the cardiac monitor on the bed next to the patient. I heard Nickie give a slight chuckle as she stepped past me, heading toward the door.

"I'll stand outside," she said.

The lieutenant, realizing what I was about to do, echoed, "Uh, me too."

I placed three EKG pasties on the patient's head, one in the center and one on each lobe. Next I attached the cable and turned on the monitor. The monitor registers electrical activity from the heart. If placed on the head, it will also register electrical activity.

Behind me I heard an EMT say, "I didn't know you could do that."

I looked over my shoulder and said, "We paramedics can do a lot."

I figured he was playing along. Once the pasties were in place, I looked at the baseline activity. Every time he moved his head, the monitor showed a big jump and beeped. The two EMTs, the patient, his daughter, and wife were focused on the screen. I hit record as he moved his head. Once I had a hard copy, I examined it intently then looked the patient.

"Sir, do you see this?" I said, pointing to the base line. He nodded his head and the machine beeped. "Sir, this baseline is normal activity."

"Praise, Jesus," yelled the wife.

"Do you know what this means?" I asked as I pointed to the aberration, a large spike on the strip.

"No," he said and the machine beeped.

"That means you have a bleed in your brain and you will be dead in the morning."

"Oh Jesus. Oh, Jesus. Please save my husband," the wife cried.

"Daddy. Oh, daddy, please don't die," the girl whimpered.

"Okay, sir, it's up to you," I said, letting it bleep a few more times.

He looked at his hysterical family pleading with him to go to the hospital. I didn't say another word, as I removed the wire cable, but left the pasties attached to his head. "Seems like you are a very rich man, loved by these two beautiful ladies. If you want them to find you dead . . ."

"Okay, I'll go. But I will walk."

"That's fine with me." So with an eruption of "Thank you, Jesus. Oh, Sweet Jesus, thank you," we got him into the back of the Basic unit and were en route to the hospital.

Once at Saint Luke's Hospital, the patient compromised and went in on a chair. As we entered, a doctor looked at the pasties on the man's head and said, "What the . . ."

"Go back to what you were doing doctor, I'll triage," said Bill, a male nurse.

"Okay, what's up?" said Bill, as he saw us grinning. He was used to our antics aimed at doing right by the patient. Perhaps our methods were a bit unorthodox, but they worked.

That night I explained, "The electro-brain scan confirmed a basilar skull fracture." I noticed two doctors now listening intently. "The gentleman was knocked unconscious with a large piece of wood, has positive nausea, vomiting, and battle signs behind his ear. He would not accept the long board or collar. He did not want to talk to our doctors or come here until we confirmed the bleed with our Life Pack 5."

"Great. Get him into that bed," Bill said, pointing to the crash room.

As Nickie and I walked out to get our equipment, I heard the two doctors ask Bill, "Who are they and what was that all about?"

"Those two, the guy talking and the girl are New York City paramedics. As to what it's all about? They just saved a man's life."

Sure enough, because of the good work of the EMTs and a little good old "waking hypnosis," the man was taken up to the operating room.

Outside, the good lieutenant called me off to the side as Nickie stowed some gear.

"Hey Jim, nice going. Nickie and I almost busted our guts, but you need to do me a favor." For this EMS boss, the world.

"Sure, what's up?"

"Those two EMTs actually believed that you could do a brain scan with the cardiac monitor. Clue them in, please."

With this, he started laughing.

"No, they . . ." I started to say and then recalled the one's statement, "Gee, I didn't know you could do that." I looked at him and started to laugh. I couldn't wait to tell Nickie. I told her and we walked over to the two EMTs doing their paperwork.

"Nice going, guys." Both smiled. "So you really enjoyed what we did with the monitor, huh?"

"Oh yeah, it was . . ." We knew we had them.

"Oh, no. We knew you were playing all the time."

We had them cold. To help ease their pain, I said over my shoulder as we were leaving, "Hey, the name of the game is to get them to the hospital. We are the patient's advocate and sometimes it's the patient, not the doctor that needs the convincing."

One of those EMTs was Kevin Kane. He later became a firefighter and died on March 5, 1991 serving with Ladder Company 110. Our crews brought him in, equipment melted to his body. He gave his life searching an abandoned building for homeless people reportedly trapped in the inferno; there were none.

Sometimes, you have to get involved because it's the right thing to do.

One night, Nickie and I were going up Broadway when we saw a black male about six feet tall run from a building, go into a military stance behind a car, and point a black service revolver at the entrance to the building. I proceeded up Broadway to the light.

"Jimmy, did you see that?" she asked with her cute English accent.

"Yep," I responded, knowing what this gutsy lady was thinking. But I waited to hear her say it.

"We have to do something, Jimmy." I smiled as I made a U-turn facing south with a visual of the perp.

"Get out of the seat belt, get on the floor, and call for a sector," I told her, figuring perhaps the perp would fire on us.

"Paramedics to Central," Nickie said, calling the police dispatcher.

"Paramedic?" the police dispatcher came back.

"We are at . . . ," there was a pause when she looked up from the floor asking, "where the fuck are we?" Now it was an agitated English accent, but still cute. I gave her the location, giggling to myself. She gave the location, and continued, "We have a black male in his teens wearing dark pants and a light, short-sleeve shirt, with a handgun, on the east side of the street." As we stood by, the sector responded. But as they came northbound on Broadway, the perp spotted them. He darted across to the west side of the tree-lined island that divided Broadway. He sat on the chain fence, camouflaged by the shadows, trees, and shrubs. I watched in horror. As the two cops pulled up, looking east at the entrance to the building, the perp raised his weapon.

"Oh shit," I said.

"What?" Nickie asked, as I stepped on the gas, throwing on the lights and siren. As we accelerated, I told her that under no circumstances was she to get up. I passed the perp and locked up the brakes, coming to a jarring halt several feet past him.

I threw open the door, jumping clear of the vehicle, and screamed at him, "Do you know where 250 is?" With total surprise and confusion, he lowered the weapon, offering me time to take a few more steps. Once close enough I tackled him. The cops realized what happened and came running, guns drawn. My partner was out of the vehicle in case I needed some support.

An EMS lieutenant who was monitoring the frequency came over. He was the ass wipe who dropped the dime to Hawk Eye concerning Barry Travis and me years ago at King's County. He was now an officer. For five minutes I listened to this dip jump up and down, "It's not your job. You are not cops. You should have only reported it and not gotten involved. I'm trying hard not to have you brought up on charges, Schrang."

Well, at least this ass wipe remembered my name. Tactically, I did everything correctly. I have had similar experiences in other parts of the world. I kept track of the perp and moved the vehicle past the kill zone to protect my partner from a shot. I also employed the element of surprise to take him down. It pays to not only to hear, but to listen.

I asked him, "So you would rather we let two cops get shot then work on them?"

He replied, "That's your job." That said it all. Nickie tried to intercede several times, but he cut her off, glaring at me. She stood dumfounded with her cute mouth open after hearing his final statement. I heard this ass wipe who had carried around his gutless act all these years and was now getting revenge. I heard a lieutenant who would have to answer to the gods, if I got hurt. If that happened, the dirty little secret that our job was dangerous would get out to the public. The mayor's office wouldn't allow that. When he was done, I got back into the vehicle, shaking my head. Lieutenant or not, *Jonathan* was still a spineless loser.

So you think priests are the only ones who deal with entities from other worlds?

That same night, we were assigned an "Altered Mental Status" further up town. Nickie and I felt refreshed to leave the loser's area of operation and get a job in Dominican Land. We pulled up, unloaded our gear, and climbed the stairway, entering the gloomy lobby of the building. Standing on one side of the door, radio turned down, I knocked.

"Come in," came a strange and eerie voice from within the apartment. We both looked at each other.

"You come to the door, please," I requested, not having a good feeling.

"I can't. You need to help me," came the response.

I forcefully pushed the door open. There was a wall in front of me with a long hallway going to the right, which was dimly lit. To the left was the living room.

"I'm here," went the voice, coming from the living room. I watched the hallway as we entered. The living room was well lit. The patient, a male Hispanic about sixty, was seated on a long couch. A large stove and sink were in the same room to his right. I wondered about this strange layout.

"How can we help you, sir?" I asked, surveying the apartment.

Nickie stood to his left, her back to the kitchen area. He looked at her and licked his lips. His cream-colored skin was wrinkled and dry.

"Hey, hello! Look at me, please. My partner is already spoken for."

He swiveled his head toward me. His eyes were demonic.

"Okay, I'll try this once again. How can we help you?"

"Feed me," he hissed, staring at Nickie, before slithering off the couch, feet first! Startled, Nickie jumped back and grabbed a big, heavy, frying pan. As the guy continued to slither onto the floor, I looked at her.

"What are you doing?" I asked, laughing.

In total seriousness she responded, "Defending you!"

"Thanks, Nickie, but how about calling for a sector and seeing where our backup is?"

"Okay," she said, "but I'm standing over here." She headed for the door. It was really a remarkable scene. Nickie, beautiful as ever, her blue eyes flashing, talked on the portable radio, holding a frying pan. The patient continued to slither and hiss, just like a snake. Help arrived and we had to secure the patient since he attempted to bite as we took him out.

The PRU was history and we were moved back into the buses.

Not all of my partners had the class, personality, maturity, integrity, or spirit of Nickie. But there were three other great paramedics: Carlos Nuñez, Joe Hodak, and Simeon Klebner.

One morning, Carlos Nuñez and I were ready to go home when we received a call for a "Difficult Breather." We arrived to find the patient going into acute pulmonary edema (APE), and she had forgotten to take her water pills for several days.

We started our dance. Carlos placed the high-concentration, non-rebreather oxygen mask over her wet face and confirmed what we already knew. Her lungs were filling up with fluid. Meanwhile, I got her blood pressure, pulse, and a fast EKG strip, holding the cheap pasties on the patient.

She answered Carlos's questions and complained of chest pain radiating to her right scapular and jaw. I gave her an 81 mg baby aspirin, as mandated by EMS gods, even though hospital staff members complained because we did not give adult dosages. I started the IV and pushed the Lasix, a water pill in liquid form. Its purpose was to get fluid back where it belonged and have the patient urinate the rest. The main effect was to eliminate excess fluid.

While I waited, I placed a nitroglycerin pill under her tongue to dilate and open the vessels and decrease the load on the heart. Carlos called to clear for the use of Lasix and morphine.

In those days we were supposed to wait until the doctor cleared the Lasix. The reality was paramedics would give everything short of the narcotics and then call. We were supposed to be a team, but when the doctors realized we were doing the right things, they gave clearance at our discretion. The patient received the life-saving medication without delay. This was what teamwork was about.

By the time we moved the patient into the chair for the trip to the hospital, she felt great. The EKG strip cleared up. Her breathing was better. The chest pain was gone and her pressure was fine.

That morning, the patient was blessed to have Dr. Sheridian at telemetry. This man was a team player, a gentleman, not an ego-oriented doctor. This was not the case with the majority. The husband and wife sang our praises and asked if we wanted them to send letters to the mayor or our bosses. We explained it was unnecessary and that it was our pleasure to help.

Back at Bellevue, I had started to re-stock when Carlos came over and told me, "We have a problem."

Automatically, when anyone said to me, "We have a problem," it translated to "I, James M. Schrang, have a problem."

"I was so tired, I forgot to ask for the morphine."

"No problem, let me call telemetry," I said, not really giving it much thought. I just finished the tour with a competent, hardworking paramedic, who was busting his ass in school. He was studying to be a nurse. Big deal a mistake was made; nevertheless, it was the right drug, right dosage, right patient, right route, given at the right time. I finished what I was doing, then called telemetry at Puzzle Palace. Telemetry was a closet at Maspeth where we called in to get orders or to have a medical consult. First we'd talk to a paramedic, who screened the call, and then to the doctor. Most paramedics at telemetry were cool.

First I talked to Dr. Sheridian, who agreed with the treatment and had no problem with it. I'd have to talk to our boss, the floor lieutenant, to get a narcotics number.

"Hi boss. This is paramedic Jim Schrang. I just spoke to Dr. Sheridian, who cleared us to ask you for a narcotics number for the last call."

"You have a problem, Schrang. You're out of morphine."

"No, I don't have the problem, EMS has the problem. Besides, I'm not out of morphine. I never touch the stuff."

"You are not getting a number."

"Hey, the doctor cleared it. You're a lieutenant, he is the doctor."

This was going from bad to worse, but I didn't see the connection yet.

"When was the last time you were in the street and accidentally made a mistake?" I asked.

"Listen here, son . . ." Oh cool, now I'm his son.

This was going nowhere so I responded, "Son? No you listen to this." Slam. I hung up on the fool.

I still did not believe we had a problem, just a misguided officer's ego attempt to act self-important. I went upstairs to see Chief Ionerelli. I explained the situation to him. He chuckled at the stupidity of the lieutenant trying to overrule the doctor. Then the phone rang. Dr. Barbara

Macintosh was the Medical Director, Lorraine Giordano's assistant. She said we were restricted patient care.

I later learned that the lieutenant went upstairs, screaming, "Schrang is giving morphine out for free." This was where everything tied in.

A week and a half earlier paramedic Joe Hodak and I had a critical, combative APE in the lobby of a hotel. As usual, the Roosevelt paramedic unit didn't pick up their job, so we traveled a distance to help the patient. Now Joe, aside from being in commercials on TV with his twin brother, was also a great paramedic, who would give you the shirt off his back. He called for the morphine and got Dr. Crisari, who was not known for his team-playing spirit. Dr. Crisari, on several occasions, had been just plain rude and egotistical on the phone. That night we desperately needed the morphine and we were denied it in an unprofessional manner, according to Joe. We packaged the patient and ran to Roosevelt Hospital, where the doctors laid into us for not giving the morphine.

Joe felt so outraged, he decided to write up Dr. Crisari. I knew it was pointless, but he was my partner, and above all, a friend. I felt a restrained rage that the patient didn't receive what he was supposed to, but I'd seen it happen with these doctors before. An M.D. can be a license to kill, and nothing happens to the doctor. The letter went forward, with a supporting statement from me. Of course nothing happened then, but it was about to.

Several days later, we were ordered to report to Dr. Giordano's office. Carlos had taken the family to Disney World and would arrive a little later. Dr. Macintosh called me into the office. Carlos wasn't missing anything, since I watched as the EMS version of Disney World began here. Dr. Giordano sat behind her desk. I was asked what happened and Dr. Macintosh listened intently. Finally, Dr. Macintosh showed her colors.

"Remember you work under my license."

"No, I work under Dr. Giordano's license. Remember she, not you, is the boss." I could tell from the tone and statements where this was going. The best defense was a good offense, so I said to Dr. Macintosh, "This is all about the letter Joe wrote and I co-signed, right?"

"I listened to the tape and Dr. Crisari did the right thing."

"Not according to the doctors at Roosevelt Hospital." I retorted.

Agitated, she relied, "He's a doctor." Oh good, when all else fails let's hide behind titles and the hell with patient care.

"Listen, *doctor*," I responded, staring at her, "you can have all the ego you want in medicine. But when it comes to healing, it's a team effort and there is no ego."

With this, she got up and left as abruptly as she had entered.

Dr. Giordano looked at me and said, "You had better watch yourself out there."

"Doctor, you have never heard me curse once, even when you suspended me for going to Bosnia." I had gone on humanitarian and medical relief missions to Bosnia, walking the streets and treating people who were hit by Serbian rocket and rifle fire. "However," I continued, "what the hell am I supposed to do if I can't trust my partner? Am I supposed to use a tape?" She didn't reply. There was a knock on the door and Carlos walked in.

"So, I've heard Jim's version. What is your version?" she asked.

"It's all Jim's fault." Carlos said.

I looked at the doctor and said, "See, I've been telling you it's my fault."

Carlos laughed and said, "No really, it's my fault. I was tired and thought I had asked for the morphine."

We were told, "Okay, accidents happen. Both of you are back to duty." We left.

Within three weeks, a paramedic who worked in the Medical Director's Office did some overtime with another paramedic. In one night, two separate patients were given the wrong narcotic. Not a damn thing happened of consequence. It seems that Dr. Macintosh didn't feel it was a big thing. Later the paramedic became a lieutenant. Does this sound like discrimination? It sure as hell does, but it gets better.

Let's go back to the streets for a breath of fresh air.

One day Simeon Klebner and I were given an "Unconscious" call on the yuppie Eastside of Manhattan. Among the gigantic concrete and steel skyscrapers lives the upper crust of, not only America, the world. These are the movers and shakers. Their mansions reach the sky. Their egos float just as high, separated from reality of the earth and lost in their self-importance. In this part of Manhattan, the rich and famous live, shop, and play.

On this overcast day, we pulled up to a well-known restaurant seen in magazines and on TV. The call was not inside the yuppie hangout, but at the corner bus stop. Huddled under a dark green plastic bag sat a young, black man.

"Yo man, what's happening?" No answer.

Simeon asked, "What's your name, man?" The young man looked at us. He was in his late twenties. Already his black nappy hair had hints of gray in it. His face was thin and his eyes showed the price of the streets. I saw brown baggy pants from under the bag protecting his legs. He wore no socks, just old, black shoes.

"Buy me a cheeseburger and I'll tell you," was his reply. Simeon looked at me and we both smiled. I reached in my pocket and we pooled our money.

Just then, the "Embassy Guards" of the Nineteenth Precinct pulled up. They had all the various embassies in their precinct. On a number of occasions they had been too forceful with the homeless. They definitely lacked the street smarts, or caring, of cops in ghetto areas.

As we stepped from Stress Free, they pulled up beside the young man. He sat in silent resignation as the Embassy Guards asked, "Want us to take care of this?"

This? I thought to myself.

In unison both of us responded, "No, we can take care of this." They drove off, never realizing how we just mocked their ignorance. However, this inflection was not to fall on deaf ears. Simeon went inside to place the order as I squatted down by the young man.

"What are you doing out here?"

He realized we were not going to hurt him, as he'd been so often hurt before, and said, "Listen, man, my name is William. I'm not hurting anyone. I'm afraid to sleep in the shelters or even Central Park. All I'm doing is begging for money to eat. I don't hurt no one."

I could understand his fear of not wanting to sleep in a shelter. The one across from Columbia Presbyterian Hospital at 168th Street was a virtual war zone, a sea of broken humanity. The sergeant from the Thirty-fourth Precinct had to draw his gun and put it to the head of the administrator to get him, his partner, and the EMS crew out safely. The staff at these facilities incited racial conflicts and preyed on and accepted "donations" from the residents.

Aside from the fear this man would have of being raped, he would also be exposing himself to the super tuberculosis strains rampant in these facilities. All of our liberal-minded yuppies were concerned about civil violations against citizens. This was all fine and good.

But TB was a case where the welfare of the majority should preclude the rights of the offender. We'd bring a homeless person to the hospital and the staff would start them on medications for TB. For whatever reason, drugs, alcohol, lack of education or mental illness, once released, the person would not complete treatment. Thus the TB grew resistant to the medications if and when the individual was brought to the hospital again. This man had much to fear.

As we spoke, I wondered what the road he traveled had taught him. He was articulate, yet not part of society. He was rich in experiences and was a symbol, reminding society of its role in humanity. Stepping out of society was not a disadvantage, but being segregated from it was.

"It's ready, Jim," called Simeon, looking at me.

"We'll be right there, Sim," I said, noting a big smile on Simeon's face. We both knew what we needed to do here to show this man dignity and put the owners of the restaurant in their place.

There was no "unconscious." But it was bad business to have this beggar in front of the posh restaurant. The sanitation department couldn't dispose of this "human garbage," but EMS could remove it. Simeon and I knew what the deal was.

"Okay, William, your cheeseburger is ready. Let's get that bag off and go inside to eat."

Shock raced across his face as he gasped, "I can't go in there. They don't want me. I'm black."

"Yeah, we kind of realize you're black. We paramedics can pick up things like that," I said with a smile. He looked confused and scared. "But the bottom line is that you are a man. Thus we are going inside, so let's go." He stood up, folded his garbage bag, and we proceeded into the restaurant. As I held the door for him, there was a blond beauty facing us.

I heard her ask the boyfriend, "What are they doing with him?"

"They are probably buying him something and then they will leave," he confidently responded.

After hearing that remark, I took a table next to this charming couple. Talk about burying their heads in the sand. Simeon brought over the meal and fast on his heels was the Greek manager.

"You can't stay here," he yelled.

"Excuse me. Who are you talking to?" I asked, looking around the chic restaurant.

"Him. He can't stay here."

"Oh, you mean William?"

"Yes."

"Well, William's meal is paid for. And William will eat it in your restaurant," I said. Flabbergasted, he looked at me with hatred and rage.

"I want him and you out!"

"Wrong," I said in a controlled tone. I recalled what Sun Tzu, a Chinese warrior genius, taught in *The Art of War*. Anger and greed are fundamental in defeat. An unemotional, calm warrior will be the victor. This guy was the epitome of anger and greed.

"How long have you been in America?"

Totally confused, he answered, "Ten years. What does this have—"

Before he could finish, I raised my hand and he stopped talking. Again in a controlled monotone voice, "William here is an American. As such, he has money, has ordered a meal, and has every right to eat the meal you are serving him."

The guy stood silent. I decided to go for the kill. William hadn't started eating yet, as he sat, looked and listened. Simeon stood behind the guy with a bright grin on his face. "Now, here is what is going to take place. William will finish his meal in peace. After he is done, if he wishes to use the restroom, he shall, then leave. If under any circumstances we get a call back here from William, we, Stress Free Paramedics, will shut you down." The guy's mouth hit the floor, but I wasn't finished. "We paramedics will issue you health and safety violations, closing you down until the hearing. Am I making this perfectly clear to you?" The guy nodded. "Fine, now I'm sure you are needed elsewhere in this fine establishment. So please excuse us while we do the paperwork."

Simeon sat down. With the aisle clear, the two yuppies didn't miss a beat, since William was ripe. As he launched into his meal, they launched as fast as their legs would carry them, out the door. Between chews, William gave us the information we needed to complete our paperwork. Simeon nodded and I looked out the window. Little miss yuppie gagged, then vomited, as the macho boyfriend held her. Both cleared the area. It must have been the food.

With the paperwork done, we ordered and waited till another soda and French fries were delivered to William. We left William engrossed in his meal. As I walked to the counter, I reminded the proprietor, "Goodbye, sir. Remember what I said." He nodded.

To confirm it, Simeon called, "See, William. Remember, if you need us, call for Stress Free One Oh Zee." William smiled, waved, and went back to eating his feast.

As we pulled away, I did a high five. Once again we fought for freedom. I never received an "Unconscious" call on that corner again.

FOUR

Fidney Paupers
— or —
The Twilight of the Gods

Gods ruled by fear, but now it was they who were afraid.
—Xena, in an episode of *Princess Warrior*

The Fire God, FDNY Commissioner Thomas Von Essen, having his own uniformed gods, no longer needed the lesser, civilian gods. On January 5, 1998, the Bureau of EMS was reduced to EMS Command, without even a whimper. EMS chiefs lost all their power.

Fear is the loss of power and control. In reality it is False Evidence Appearing Real.

The chiefs created the myth of their paramilitary organization, the notion of their self-importance. They substituted fear for good management skills, education, and leadership. These myths were as superficial and as shallow as they were. They never learned that highly functional people have no desire or investment in controlling people. What they projected and made their reality came back to them, as is the universal law of Creation.

On March 17, 1996, EMS had been given to the fire department to justify its existence. It was a political payoff by Mayor Rudolph Giuliani. Thomas Von Essen, who had been the head of the fire department's union, became commissioner of the fire department for endorsing Giuliani in his mayoral bid against David Dinkins. MetroCare president, Steve Zakheim, who had contributed substantial funds to the Giuliani campaign, wanted his payoff. His reward was the go-ahead for a for-profit ambulance service in 911. Yes, Rudy paid well. But at what cost to the people?

After years of rumors of drug and alcohol abuse, rape, and illiterate, yes illiterate EMS chiefs, it was all coming home to roost. Listen to the answer given on national TV during a major snowstorm by the Chief in Charge of NYC EMS, David Diggs. When asked if there was a plan to deal with the snowstorm emergency, Mr. David Diggs stated, "We have a plan for a plan." Talk about not being the brightest bulb in the marquee!

I was at the academy for a refresher when the then mayor, all self-important Mayor Ed Koch, gave a speech in front of a graduating class of new EMTs. He stood there for a moment. His arrogance was exceeded only by his illusion of self-importance.

Then he stated, "Now you can use EMS as a stepping stone to become nurses, firefighters . . ." If that was not bad enough, he continued, "You people are only file clerks in ambulances." Not one chief said a word in defense of EMS and its valuable service or potential career path.

Some chiefs asked good-looking EMTs to be their "aides" on the midnight tours. They engaged in extramarital affairs, resulting in rumors and questions about paternity. There were lesbian affairs of a clique that would have made the "Teflon Don," John Gotti, proud.

I held no maliciousness toward others who were not heterosexual. In fact, I considered the life style to be exactly that, a life style chosen by a soul to experience. I considered all life styles to be equal in nature.

What I did have a problem with was when a clique, no matter what the label, was obsessed with power. This clique became tyrannical, employing intimidation and subversion to gain control of people and of positions. The clique's tentacles extended from the Office of Medical Administrator to other administrative titles within Health and Hospital Corporation, to include, but not limited to, the CCU.

One sordid incident of jilted love resulted in the arrest and humiliation of a beloved, respected captain. The captain was a credit to the service and a pleasure to work with. The arrest involved Dr. Macintosh as a key player sitting in OMA (Office of Medical Administrator) when the captain was cuffed, in uniform, at her station, in full view of her people. As this occurred, our Medical Director, Dr. Lorraine Giordano, was mute. Certain chiefs just chuckled and Dr. Macintosh got the nickname of "Dr. Bob" on the streets by the less-than-amused paramedics. No one took responsibility for allowing the clique to target an individual or conduct character assassinations.

In an incident involving repeated sexual abuse by a male officer, one female paramedic was awarded more than a million dollars. In another case, a female paramedic had a female lieutenant transferred out of the borough because of sexual harassment.

The same lieutenant was on duty one night at Bellevue when a large sum of money, collected to help a member, disappeared. She was still at Bellevue when a large snow blower disappeared. The lieutenant was next moved to Metropolitan. There she and her lover created problems for a female paramedic. The female paramedic, who was a very competent lady, threatened the gods with a lawsuit. Because of this, and only this, the lieutenant in question was moved once again.

Now at a Bronx command, a male officer, a cross-dresser himself, found two crates of oxygen bottles missing after the newly transferred lieutenant's tour. Seems she also worked at a for-profit ambulance service.

The EMS officer who found the cases of oxygen bottles missing was transferred after he revealed that several voluntary units were not doing the correct thing. His report would have reflected badly on Mayor Giuliani and Fire Department Commissioner T. Von Essen, thus bringing more heat to the EMS chief's shrinking world.

There were other signs of abuse and corruption. A weapon was reportedly found in a chief's car. There were rumors of cell phone use to call 900 numbers for sex. The chiefs claimed no conflict of interest when they ran the Borough of Manhattan, yet worked as paramedics at the Javitts Center, which was contracted out to Saint Vincent's Hospital, a voluntary hospital in the 911 system. Yeah, right.

One lieutenant from the Bellevue station spent more than a year documenting abuses by Cabrini units. When the lieutenant attempted to forward the report, he was ordered to back off by a chief who was attempting to take over the Cabrini ambulance department. When the report was leaked, it caused an uproar. The chief retired back into the security of the gods.

Management's inability to run the world's largest EMS system took its toll. They showed their true colors with their gutless sellout to the merger in front of the city council. In one moment of destiny, they had the opportunity to redeem themselves, defend themselves, and make the merger profitable for both FD and EMS. The chiefs needed a viable union presence for our members to galvanize and present an organized front to the fire department. Such an effort could have resulted in EMS leadership. In particular, the crews and the people we served could have gained much. The result would have deflated the Fire God. But it was a risk no one would take, since each feared for his own survival. So the implosion began.

Even the chiefs who had always been the icons of hope—Robert Ionerelli, Joel Friedman, Gustav Papas—became silent observers, cowering to the dictates of a force they never fathomed. The Fire God had an insatiable appetite.

A mover and shaker, Chief Paul Maniscalco would be the first casualty in opposing the Fire God. His arrogance and self-importance would lead to his downfall.

Knowledge was pointless if one couldn't communicate it in a useful form to the weakest link in the chain. The chain was made up of weak, and in some cases, useless buffoons. Yet, Maniscalco was an EMS professional when it came to his vision of the service. We would not be the bastard children of the Health and Hospital Corporation and now the fire department. Those chiefs like Maniscalco, Ionerelli, Friedman, Pappas, and a few others who wished to learn and make the job better were the minority. The inept, gutless pencil-pushing pukes were the majority.

Thanks to years of Becker's "leading by fear," the weaker ones were only interested in hearing their own godly commands. By their actions, even the ones with potential relinquished their sacred role to provide leadership and the best care for our public. Instead of admitting we were given to the fire department to justify its existence as a political payback to Mayor Guiliani, they folded, cowered, and sang the Fire God's praises.

We medics watched repeatedly as the fire engines responded a minute to a minute and a half before we received the cardiac jobs. We complained and we were ignored. The public suffered and people died just so the mayor and fire commissioner could say their program was working.

The chiefs had never learned of the Native American belief, "No tree has branches so foolish as to fight among themselves." The implosion continued. Some EMS chiefs, after trying to debunk the current chief in charge, bailed out, and went to OEM, Office of Emergency Management. One told us, "I'm still one of you guys," not realizing that he could never be one of us. We still owned our souls.

Another chief tried to make points with the mayor by designing a disaster plan for MetroCare, the mayor's for-profit, politically bought ambulance service, or as we called it, "Rudy's EMS."

In February of 1998, the paramedic units received Atropine and 2Pam kits for a chemical attack. Next the chiefs' cars, as if they could be counted on to back us up in an emergency, received them. Finally, and much later, the Basic units were issued Atropine and 2Pam kits. The federal government had informed us, New York City would get hit with it. The 1992 bombing of the World Trade Center had been a wake-up call for the federal government, but not for our gods.

With the distribution of the kits, we requested gas masks. The request fell on deaf ears in the Medical Director's Office. Doctors jockeyed for position, cutting each other's throats to appear as the golden choice to the Fire God.

To quell any fear, a chief came to our station to disclose that Dr. Dario

Gonzales had set up the plan for such an incident and that we, the EMS crews, would be in the "Cold Zone." This came from a doctor who had never seen combat. We learned some information from medical students entering the EMS fellowship program. They told us of his derogatory remarks about the paramedics. This was from a man who went out to the federal building explosion, never recovered a body, but reportedly was traumatically affected by what he saw.

Evidently, his experience didn't translate into common sense or concern for EMS crews within his responsibility. He didn't read *The Art of War* by Sun Tzu or realize that combat is fluid in nature, not static like firehouse mentality.

Instead, he had a dog and pony show at Bellevue, ground zero. The EMS instructors told us the truth. It was a ploy to appease us, and the casualties would be high. In fact, the gods already accepted massive EMS losses, which was totally unacceptable to combat veterans like paramedic Lou Cook and myself.

An EMT asked the chief, "What happens if we are at ground zero, in a cold zone, and the wind shifts?"

"You'll be dead," he said in a cold, unemotional voice. When we asked again about protective masks, we were told none would be coming. From the chemical attack in Japan, they had learned about off-gassing and put it to good use. The chiefs reportedly had a computer model to show how many trips an unprotected EMT could make to the hospital, ambulance loaded with casualties, before he was overcome by the off gases.

After much research, Lou Cook and I got the specs for the gas masks and filters we wanted, and the search was on. I went to Samgong Industrial Company in Seoul, Korea. Their GM (Gas Mask)-148K with K-1 canister was just the item we needed. Then I adapted an American chemical-biological hood. Numerous delays followed.

Chief Robert McCracken, then in charge of the EMS Bureau, met with us on August 13, 1998 at Battalion Eight, Kips Bay Station in Bellevue. The meeting had been put off several times because the chief had to attend local community board meetings, showing where his priority was.

Below is an excerpt of a letter I sent Chief Robert McCracken on August 17, 1998. It says a lot about the mentality of the civilian chiefs of EMS as well as the Fire God.

> It should be brought to your attention that the lackluster program which paramedics were given, as directed by Dr. Gonzales to satisfy a federal mandate, was not in compliance with federal guidelines, nor did it demonstrate any sound combat logic. To reiterate, we have been told that Fire Suppression, (Firemen) as well as our ERS (Emergency Response Squad, glorified HazTac) crews will be in protective gear. We (EMTs and Paramedics) will be in the Warm Zone. We will not be wearing protective gear or have escape hoods available because Dr. Gonzales has 'Drawn the Circles.' The thinking is non-combat wishful thinking by the politically correct. It will deplete our resources and increase casualties of our EMS crews. It will make nil our ability to protect the Fire Suppression and ERS Teams in the Hot Zone or serve the public. Instead it will aid and serve said terrorists in their attempt to inflict maximum casualties with minimum loss to their side. This mentality, is also in direct violation of Janes Chem-Bio Handbook. Endorsed by Mayor Rudolph Guiliani, Howard Safir, Commissioner NYPD, Jerome Hauer, Director, Mayors Office of Emergency Management and Thomas Von Essen, Commissioner, NYFD, as our guidelines for such terrorist attack. It is a doctrine supported by our military, as they are the supporting co-authors.

I explained why I had decided on the GM-148K with K-1 canister with the adaptation of the chemical bio hood standard with the United States Army. The result of this letter was interesting.

Deputy Chief Randy Hirth had asked me about the masks, but he never gave me a hard time about them. I have worked several MCIs (Mass Casualty Incidents) with him and his aide, Grace Cacciola. I honestly cannot think of a single time I had a problem with the way either one conducted an operation. He was always supportive of his people. All he required was we do our jobs.

This was not the case with Division Commander Pedro Carrasquillo.

During my meeting with Chief McCracken, I voiced my belief that Division Commander Carrasquillo had repeatedly demonstrated his inability to be effective and to appreciate that Manhattan was target-rich for a terrorist strike. His demonstrated inability to logically answer why EMS medic units were changed at a whim or why it appeared the voluntary units got the better hours. He had an inept statement, "You are assigned a tour." That was not an answer.

After my meeting with Chief McCracken, I had another shipment of masks on the way, since more people wanted to buy them. At Bellevue, the chief asked me, "By whose authority are you carrying that? Who knows about this? Who is sanctioning this? Is the union aware of this?"

Paramedic Tom Reynolds laughed as I said, "Let's see how long it takes before he starts trouble."

One week later, paramedic Lou Cook was summoned downtown and grilled about the masks. Then Chief Carrasquillo called the desk at Bellevue. Lieutenant JoAnn Kovac received the call. The chief was ordering her to tell everyone, "Masks are not to be on the units whether they are personal safety items or not. They are not issued by FD."

Then Lieutenant Kovac informed him, "Chief, if you are still standing after this is over, you can write me up." He went ballistic.

"How many masks do you have?"

"I always carry one."

"Expect a call from Captain Charlie Wells ERS (Emergency Response Squad)."

That evening, Captain Phil Para saw me in the emergency room at Bellevue. "Oh, so you are the guy selling these?" As if he didn't know. He worked down at Station Eleven with the Borough Office (The Enchanted Forest) where Chief Carrasquillo resided.

"I think I'll get one. Can I see yours?" A discussion followed and I gave him the information. He knew the date of the next shipment, country of origin, and the like. I saw it all coming and was letting it happen, because as usual I was one step ahead of these amateurs. Dear old Pedro and the rest of the gang were spending a lot of energy to ensure our people weren't protected. If half of this energy was expended ensuring the safety of EMTs and paramedics, we would stand a fighting chance. But that was not EMS supervision. Whatever their move, I knew I could and would beat it.

As expected, they made their move. Or was it coincidence again? On April 23, 1998, a week after my little talk with Captain Para, I received a phone call from a customs agent at JFK International Airport.

He told me, "You have to come over and sign a form so the shipment can be released."

"Any problem?" I asked.

"Oh no. You need to sign a form and you'll have your items."

I went over in my little fire department superman outfit and took them by surprise. I cordially mixed in and walked through the so-called security. I stood in front of the desk and as the agent spoke on the phone, I waited for him to hang up. I introduced myself and actually startled him.

"How did you get through security?" he demanded.

"By my good looks."

When he had regained his composure, I asked about the form and I took out my pen. I realized there was more to the game.

"Please wait in this office and I'll be there in a moment."

I found myself in an interrogation room. I looked around and waited for the next act. Three agents interrogated me. They all left a lot to be desired. I asked how these items were flagged and was told, "By the item name, gas masks."

"Cool," I said, asking, "How come my other shipment wasn't flagged?"

"The quantity of this shipment." That's funny because this was a smaller shipment.

"Who dropped the quarter? Was it Chief Carrasquillo? He is the only one giving me a hard time."

These amateurs never even said, "Who?" This blew right over him, as I confirmed what I already knew. Next they wanted to see the paperwork and my identification. They ran a computer search on me, showing I was clean. They even went over the costs, demonstrating I was not making a profit. They were having a bad day. Finally, they asked whom I worked for. I stated, Captain Mark Stone. If these wannabe interrogators wanted to be like the real ones, they would have come back at me once I said Captain Mark Stone's name.

The least they could have done was ask, "But who is Chief Carrasquillo? I thought he was your boss."

I received more information from them by their sloppy non-professional approach than they ever got from me. After I said their actions were illegal, I was released. They could find nothing, since there was nothing to find. Still, I stayed one step ahead of them. I called the station, since I had taken the day without pay, and spoke to Captain Stone. I told him to expect a phone call from customs. Sure enough, the next day when I got to work, he told me they called. They asked if I worked for him and if he knew anything about the masks.

"Sure I do. We are all waiting for them."

That was it. I contacted a licensed customs-house broker and I delivered the shipment several days later. By the way, Captain Phil Para never ordered a mask.

On April 26, 1998, Lieutenant Charlie Frazier told Paramedic Lou Cook that "if someone falls wearing the masks they will be denied LODI (Line of Duty Injury)." This was a really intelligent statement, since the only reason the crew would wear them was if their lives were threatened by a chemical or biological attack. His next statement told me why the good chief was trying to stop me. Lieutenant Frazier stated, "Fire is upset because the masks are unfitted and the crews untrained." Hello. We would not be going through this if EMS and fire were concerned for our safety.

On April 29, 1998, I made the delivery to the crews at Bellevue. Captain Charlie Wells of ERS mysteriously showed up to talk to me about the masks. He told me of the great job he'd heard I had done in Bosnia. Old news, but I guess he figured it was a way of playing to my ego.

When he finally got around to the masks he told me, "NYC has bought masks for EMS already.

"Escape masks are for EMS, not masks that let you stay and survive in a hostile environment. EMS will be in a Cold Zone. These won't be worn until ERS units tell you to 'Don and escape' since the Cold Zone is now Warm. Fire wants to know, 'Who the hell is Schrang?'

"I want a mask so I can tear it apart to find its weakness, so you don't get into trouble."

What a buddy. With his colorful background, what more could I ask for in my corner?

"I called Chief Carrasquillo and told him they were not allowed on the unit."

This final point was really interesting. I never did, nor ever will, trust Charlie Wells. He was another one with a long and colorful history. I did not ask about the good chief and his phone call to the station. Since when does a captain tell a chief in the form of an order what can or can't be done? Finally, I told the good captain I would be willing to sit in a chamber with him. He could wear his escape mask he claimed the city already bought, and I'd wear the GM-148K with K-1 canister. I would not sit there an hour, but twenty-four hours, then walk out and piss in his pocket. I believed in the equipment that much. I didn't tell him I had already given a mask with a canister to Chief McCracken, who delivered it to the Fire God's Chief Steven King of NYC Fire Safety at 9 Metro Tech. Soon Hack Hong, the representative from Samgong Industrial Co. Ltd. in South Korea, also contacted Chief King. The letter went out on August 22, 1998.

I informed the good captain that in the military, something he knows nothing about, the only form-fitted masks, so to speak, are flight crew masks. I know, since aside from being an army paratrooper, I also flew with the Air Force Reserve. Nor does the fire department fit their Scott masks. His answer was, "Well, if you have a strange face."

Concerning training, I took each person and explained the care and use of the mask and filter. In combat, like in a terrorist strike, you cannot afford to lose resources, especially foolishly. Even with escape masks, the EMTs and paramedics would become casualties. The public would lose medical crews, already a scarce resource.

I brought up immunizations. The military has them. Why not EMS? Do you know how many units in Queens respond to a "sick" on a plane landing from an international flight? I was informed that Dr. Gonzales was against it.

In closing, I will extract my final paragraph of my letter to Chief McCracken.

> Finally, there is NO CONFIDENCE at street level for EMS Management, or ERS after what they did to us at Gramercy Park.* That is why to the person, each EMT and paramedic, has refused to follow the order of Chief Carrasquillo not to carry the GM148K on their units as 'personal safety items.'

If a picture is worth a thousand words, I can refer everyone to two photos that have been disseminated worldwide. On August 8, 2000, a rush-hour bomb exploded in a busy walkway in Moscow. As Russia's EMS retrieved the wounded and dead, they wore gas masks and gloves. The other photo appeared in the *New York Times*, on September 1, 2000. It shows construction workers entering a fire department decontamination truck to be washed down after being exposed to asbestos. The firemen were at the door ready for the workers. The firemen donned gas masks and protective clothing. Next to the yellow line stands an EMS EMT. Short-sleeve shirt, no gloves, but worse, no mask. You be the judge of which EMS system is working toward being ready.

As of the writing of this book, our people were still unprotected. The city never bought the escape masks described by Captain Wells. There was talk of refurbishing the Vietnam-era masks and storing them at a central location for the transit. That sure as hell makes a lot of sense. I got back the test mask from Chief King. He never found anything wrong with it.

The only problem here lies with the fire gods and civilian gods of EMS. These politically correct ass wipes do not understand that the United States of America is at war. Unless we have a Pearl Harbor with

*Gramercy Park is located South of Bellevue Hospital. A giant steam pipe created a massive explosion killing several people. Being the second bus on the scene, I aided two workers who were burned to death. Our SOD, later ERS, with the fire department knew in the first fifteen minutes there was a massive asbestos release. They never said a word to us. Several months later we read the fire department was suing for the loss of contaminated equipment, clothing etc. Know what EMS Management did? They ordered us to bring in our clothes. They then decontaminated the buses, the same ones that so many people had been transported in long after the incident.)

the Japanese Armed Forces on surfboards at our front door, our managers will not recognize what is happening. New York City, thanks to the ineptness that festers within both the fire and EMS commands, has placed civilians at great risk. I fear for our crews.

While battling blatant, almost criminal ineptness of our superiors—I use that term advisedly—we, the crews, continued to serve the public. One call type, EDP (Extremely Disturbed Person) or, as the crews called them, "Everyday People" I always found interesting because there was indeed a story behind their actions. While working Queens on overtime I met such an individual; in fact it turned out she was a friend of a friend. Below I have recreated her story as told to me by Helen several years ago to demonstrate the tentacles of insanity are far reaching and not only confined to the ghetto of East New York Brooklyn, but also in cupcake Queens.

Helen was eleven years old and lived with two brothers and her mother and father in a middle-class section of Queens. Her younger brother, nine-year-old Tommy, adored her. It seemed like everywhere she went he followed. Bobby was their fifteen-year-old brother. He hung out with the wrong crowd.

More than once, Helen consoled Bobby after their father beat him for one infraction or another. Bobby was tall and skinny. Their father had knocked out his front tooth during a scuffle. Bobby hung out with a black Jamaican crowd from another part of Queens.

Helen had seen Bobby hiding "stuff" under his coat when their father came home. One day she and Tommy were walking home from school, when they saw Bobby and his friends being chased by the cops. *He should have tried out for the track team*, she thought, smiling. She realized the cops wouldn't be able to catch him. Even Tommy, although a little shorter than she, was fast on his feet. When Tommy raced Helen in the schoolyard, he always won.

One day, at the dinner table she let it slip that Bobby had escaped the slow-footed, bumbling cops.

"I was never chased by any cops," he protested, as his father looked up from his dinner.

"Oh, yes, you were. We saw you and Willie Roberts being chased," Tommy chimed in.

Helen tried to silence Tommy by kicking him under the table. She realized her blunder, as her father made a fist of his paw-like hands. Their mother got up from the table and went to the kitchen to get him another beer. The rest was history as Bobby lay crying on his bed with a black eye.

Helen slipped into his room later. "Bobby, can I help?" she whispered. "Please, Bobby, talk to me." He rolled over. She gasped. His right eye was swollen shut with an ugly, black-and-blue golf ball-sized wound. His mouth was cut and swollen. His dirty blond hair was matted to his head with dried blood. He was a scrawny kid. Not much in the muscle department but loaded with anger.

"Get the hell out of here!"

She attempted to touch him. Exploding from the bed like a coiled snake striking its victim, Bobby grabbed her blouse while raising his right hand. Helen spun away. Her cheap white cotton blouse ripped open. Buttons and shell necklace went flying. But Bobby's anger prevailed as he threw her to the bed. Anger turned to uncontrollable rage, as he smacked her across the face several times. Hanging half on and off the bed by her throat, she was turning red, gasping, eyes wide with fright.

"I'm going to get you and Tommy for this," he hissed. Feeling his own physical pain, he let her go. Helen slid to the floor crying, finally stumbling out of his room into the room she shared with Tommy.

As Helen collapsed onto her bed crying, Tommy entered the room. Rolling her over, he saw a reddened face and cut lip. Helen surrendered, as her younger brother delicately removed her clenched hand holding the blouse closed. With her hands gently placed to the sides, Tommy carefully opened the blouse, exposing neck and naked chest. Anger rose as he observed the scratch marks on her chest and reddened neck. Reaching, he opened her clenched fist to find the remnants of the small shell necklace he had made for her in school. Helen didn't move. She looked unblinkingly into Tommy's eyes. "I'm sorry it broke, Tommy. I . . ."

Before she could finish, he gently placed his index finger over his older sister's cut mouth, then stood, and started for the door.

"I'm going to tell Dad!"

Helen bolted upright, reaching and grabbing his hand. "No. Please, Tommy!"

"But he hurt you, sis," he said. His voice filled with more hurt than anger. Helen's face was on fire.

"I know, but I'll be okay. Please don't tell," she begged. "Please, just get me a cold, wet face cloth and ice. Don't let Dad see you," she warned.

Several months later, it became evident Bobby was using and selling drugs. He had been busted by the police and, as usual, received his customary beating when their father had to bail him out. Aside from all the troubles he had at home, he was in trouble with his friends. He "lost" some drugs and they were looking to collect from him. Bobby knew it had been a stupid stunt, using the drugs to impress several of the local girls. Word got back fast to Willie, who headed the drug ring Bobby sold for.

Willie had been raised by his mother and never knew his father. He had no brothers or sisters. His mother was a large, angry woman who abused him often. She stood about five feet seven and, although not plump, had a solid body frame. Her round face seemed to be even more accented by her anger within. She wore bright red lipstick that further emphasized her pronounced large lips, making them stand out against her dark brown skin. Her oiled, jet-black hair matched her large eyelashes. She was a good-looking, solidly built woman, but her eyes were filled with rage, betrayal, and hurt.

The abuse to Willie was both verbal and physical. Even from an early age, he felt she was not beating or belittling him, but his father. Willie remembered a time when he was three years old. He was with his mother, standing at a bus stop. When it was time to get on the bus, his mother literally yanked him up by his school bag, which he wore on his back. She roughly slammed him into a seat, while she sat behind him next to an empty seat. She would not even sit next to him. As he dozed, she reached over and smacked him in his head. He sat staring straight ahead.

Willie remembered a fireman on the bus telling his mother that if he saw her hit him again he would call the cops. As he sat there he took it all in. Then she claimed it was their stop and yanked him off the bus. How much he wanted to stay with the fireman. How much he wanted to tell the man she hurt him. His stomach still hurt from the boiling water that she poured on him one night when he soiled himself. But Willie couldn't speak. He couldn't cry or feel pain.

Years later a woman's body was found. The EMS crew was responding to an "Unconscious" on a rooftop in a housing project. They found a headless, nude body on the hot asphalt roof. Her arms and legs were spread. Between her legs was a Shaffer beer can. Chicken feathers were sticking out of her vagina. Burn marks from a cigarette as well as hot wax were found all over the body. It appeared that her arms and feet had been tied and burned with some type of electrical wire. Her head was never found. The victim had been slowly tortured and then decapitated, with almost surgical precision. An occult religious group was blamed for the murder. There never was a conviction, nor positive identification.

Willie made money by hustling and selling drugs. He established his reputation by unleashing a fanatical, an almost demonic, degree of violence on his victims. He relished in using its excess to create unimag-. inable pain, especially to girls and older women.

Bobby was on his unkempt bed one night with the window open. A soft summer breeze swept through the window. He was in a mental haze from all the drugs. Suddenly he felt a nudge. Was this nudge real or was he imagining it? It felt real. Then it happened again. He opened his eyes to see a grotesque, masked figure over him with a large machete. The mask was in the form of a deer or elk, but it was distorted and evil looking. Black with white marks adorned the cheeks with small, sharp, discolored teeth. At the top were small antlers. The figure wore black, probably a jump suit.

Bobby wanted to scream, but his reactions were slow. A wet, filthy cloth was shoved in his mouth. Several unseen hands held him to his bed as he gagged and thrashed clumsily. Was this a nightmare?

"Listen, Bobby," said the mask, distorted as if from hell. He shook his head to make sense of what he heard, "It's your turn to pay, nigger."

He looked in horror as a dark machete was placed next to his chest. Struggling, he felt it burn as the machete slowly sliced superficially across his bare chest, drawing blood. Once a six-inch slash was completed, the tip of the machete was placed on the right side of the chest several inches below his armpit. Gradually he felt the tip dig in, breaking the skin, releasing life-giving blood! He attempted to recoil but couldn't, feeling the warm blood—his life—running down his side, forming small puddles on the dirty sheet. The machete stopped, as the owner realized he had Bobby's full attention. Signaling the boy to be still, he removed the wet cloth from his mouth. Bobby gasped, locked in terror, unable to move, chest burning and side aching.

The machete tip still in his side, Bobby gasped, "Please! Please. I'll do anything you want. Please let me live."

"You know, nigger, you owe me everything. But poor Bobby, you ain't got nothin', nothin' at all. You one dumb white ass nigger. So why should I let you live?"

Bobby recognized Willie's voice and the finality in it. He knew Willie induced pain on girls, thrilled at using violence, and loved money. Bobby had a solution.

"Listen, Willie, my old man is getting paid with a bonus on Friday. If you take him down, you'll clear over a grand."

"What you mean if I take him down?"

Realizing his error, as the machete was turned, Bobby responded. "Okay, okay! When I take him down, I'll give you the money."

Willie, looking through the mask, his yellow contacts illuminated by the moonlight, studied the fear in Bobby's eyes.

"Not good enough, chump."

"Okay. Okay!" he squirmed, as the machete dug deeper into his side. "I'll give you my sister!" The machete stopped moving.

"Where and when?"

"Friday morning around ten at the old church."

Willie pulled the machete from Bobby's side, grabbing him around the throat, holding the machete to his neck, motioning as the boys, gathered around the bed, pulled Bobby's dungarees off. Bobby could hardly breathe from the viselike grip. Finally, his shorts were removed. Now totally exposed, unable to move, he felt paralyzing terror. Willie released part of his grip as the boy obediently opened his mouth for the gag. The warm summer night's air had a chilling effect as it crossed his sweat-soaked body. His nostrils flared as he took deep breaths. The machete was hypnotically poised above him, dripping blood, ready to plunge it into his heart. A primordial death whimper of acceptance escaped as tear-filled eyes closed, waiting to die. The sight was priceless to Willie. Bobby's penis was now slowly being worked first by hand then orally. Shocked, he felt his hips starting to respond. Through tears he saw Willie's demented smile as the machete violently cut silently through the suffocating air. It stopped, the blade resting against his penis. The rag muffled Bobby's terrifying scream as his body shuddered then exploded in ejaculation.

"If you're lying, I'll cut your dick off and fuck you with it." Willie said, giggling with the others.

Placing a pillow over his head, all left as quietly as they entered. Bobby rolled into a fetal position, clutching his penis, crying.

On Friday morning, Bobby, uncharacteristically, offered to buy Helen an ice cream at the local store. Tommy would create a scene if he couldn't share in the new and improved generosity. Off they went, cutting across empty lots through the abandoned church, exiting through a side door. Outside, they moved along the eight-foot wooden wall, wading through waist-high grass. Stepping over garbage, they came to an opening about a hundred feet from the side exit of the church. The ice cream tasted great, cooling all on this warm summer morning. Helen beamed at Bobby.

"Bobby, I was really worried about you," Helen said, licking the ice cream cone.

"Thanks, but I've had a lot on my mind," he responded, looking at Tommy.

"Bobby, I love you so much."

He smiled. She knew she had her brother back. He even joked around with the cautious Tommy, who was now laughing up a storm.

As they started to head home, Bobby stopped about ten feet short of the entrance in the wall.

"What's the matter, Bobby?"

"Listen, I have something to do. I want you two to head home."

"Bobby, please tell me you won't get into trouble with Willie and his crowd," Helen pleaded.

Bobby reached over and tenderly caressed her face and then tugged on a braid. "Hey, I promised I was done with him, didn't I?" She nodded.

"Then where are you going?" asked Tommy. God, how Bobby hated this kid.

"I just have to meet someone and she . . . ," he stopped and smiled.

"Oh I know," said Tommy giggling.

"Okay, see you at home," Helen said as they started to take the long way home on the sidewalk.

"Hey, where are you going?"

"Oh it's such a beautiful day, I figured Tommy and I would take the long way home."

"No. You have to go through the church. Take the shortcut, so once I'm finished I can catch up to you."

"Oh, okay," Helen said, smiling, looking forward to spending more time with her newly found older brother. Bobby watched as Tommy disappeared into the opening in the fence. He looked at his watch. It was quarter to ten.

Both were happy as Tommy picked a white rose from a bush. Helen was going through the high grass when he called her. She turned around and he gave her the rose surrounded by several dandelions. Looking at Tommy, she realized she loved him so much. "I'm lucky to have a brother like you," she said, giggling, as she bent over kissing him. Walking ahead, holding the flowers, she thought, "What a perfect day."

They joked with each other as they entered the side door of the abandoned church. A fire had destroyed the ceiling and a good portion of the walls years ago. Both altar and thick railing were intact. Birds sang and made their home in the decaying, battered timber. The morning sun blazed through the empty, rotten frames of what used to be gigantic, stained-glass windows in the east wall. As the children entered laughing, they suddenly froze. There in the center of the altar stood Willie, dressed in black.

"Well, what we got here?" he asked.

Tommy grabbed Helen's hand and turned instinctively to escape the way they came in. It was blocked by one of Willie's boys. Holding Tommy's hand even tighter, Helen inched toward the east wall to make a run for it. Willie stood there, watching, waiting. His angry, ugly face scared all who saw him. Once they were directly in front of him, he raised his right hand. Two boys stepped out from behind some lumber in the shadows and grabbed the two children. Tommy broke fee and started to run. Helen screamed, as the boy pulled her by the hair toward the altar and Willie. She suddenly saw Tommy, heading toward the east wall, stop and look at her.

"Run, Tommy, run!" Helen screamed. Tommy ran back to save her. "No, run!" She watched as he was unmercifully knocked to the ground and pummelled by the bigger boys. His right hand still stretched out to her, then both heard the grotesque sickening snap, as his extended arm was broken. Howling in pain, he writhed in agony. Helen screamed, attempting to pull free from her captor, to get to Tommy. She felt the painful, violent jerk on her two braids.

"And where do you think you're going?"

"I have to help my brother, you bastard," she screamed, kicking him in his leg. He yelled, letting her go. Moving toward Tommy, she received a closed-fisted punch in the chest, sending her crashing to the floor. She couldn't breathe! Helen was dragged twelve feet from her brother. As she remained in the fetal position trying to catch her breath, strong assaulting hands pulled her thin arms above her head. The blouse was yanked over her head and used as a gag. Next the bra was ripped off, as her hands were forced behind her back and tied with it. Out of instinct, Helen unsuccessfully attempted to stay in the fetal position, as the boys continued their onslaught. Yellow shorts were pulled off, then sneakers, and socks. She spied Tommy. His shirt was gagging him. He looked at her, crying and writhing in agony. He was lying naked on the ground with his hands tied behind his back; there was pronounced deformity of his arm. Then, her panties were torn away.

The wooden floor was still cool. She felt her lip burning, as blood trickled onto the floor. She had bitten her lip without knowing it. Raising her head, she tried to see. Willie stepped off the altar toward the opening in the railing.

"Okay, bring me Mr. Tough Guy." Two boys grabbed Tommy, as he wailed in pain, the sound not well muffled by the gag.

"Get the bitch on her knees!"

Helen screamed being harshly pulled up by her braids.

"So, you think you're tough, huh?"

Tommy didn't move. Willie's yellow contacts flashed, as he reached over, tugging at the broken arm. The boy recoiled in tremendous pain, screaming. Sweat soaked his naked youthful body.

"You going to do as I say bitch, understand? Get the gag off." Tommy wanted to yell but was smacked hard. For a nine-year-old, he was putting up an unbelievable struggle. Helen could only cry and watch, praying he would do as he was told, so he wouldn't be hurt anymore. Willie looked over and sensed her prayer.

"Get the gag off the bitch. If she screams, cut her throat. I think she wants to say something to Tommy, right?" Helen mournfully nodded.

Once the gag was removed and she had her voice back, "Tommy?"

Tommy turned, seeing Helen kneeling, nude, hands tied behind her back, blood running from her mouth, clothes in disarray on the filthy floor. The soft sunlight caressed her tender body, beaming like a surreal wide light from the east, and freedom. Tommy's eyes, now clear of tears, looked into Helen's eyes as he heard her voice.

"Tommy," she said in a mature voice he had never heard before.

"Do as they say, Tommy. Do as they say."

Willie reached down and touched the boy's arm, causing him to recoil, shrieking in unbearable pain, looking at Willie.

"That's right, tough guy. You look at me and do as the little bitch tells you."

Willie undid his pants and brought out his seven-inch penis. He at-

vagina. She started to move her hips instinctively to help him. Tommy picked up the pace. Everyone was mesmerized by what was taking place. Not even the birds made a noise. It appeared that all of creation was reverently watching.

Helen could feel him growing, starting to stimulate her as uncontrolled moans now became audible. Black Jack pulled him out and directed his now hard penis into her rectum. Helen began to gyrate even more as the dance with Tommy continued, until he let out a loud moan and came. Willie had had enough. No one, not even his mother, had ever scared him in this way! Both children were brought to the area in front of the altar and made to lie down on their stomachs. Helen inched toward Tommy till she could feel him. Their feet were tied, gags replaced. Darkness enveloped them as they were blindfolded.

Willie and his gang started to leave. He turned, looking at them again. He wanted to kill them, her in particular. Willie was intimidated and terrified. He delivered a flurry of hateful kicks to both children. Turning, he wiped his eyes of the tears, put on his sunglasses, and walked toward his gang.

Helen was the first to regain consciousness. Her body was a mass of pain. She rolled over, trying to feel Tommy, but couldn't. She panicked, thinking he had left her, and urinated on herself fighting to get the blindfold off. As she tossed, she felt a lifeless mass next to her. Moving her head onto Tommy's hip, realizing she was lower, she worked her way up to his chest. She listened, straining to hear him breath. His chest rose. Squirming on the floor and using his body, she managed to get the blindfold off. Tommy just lay there. She scraped her face along the rough floor until the gag came free, attempting to scream, but couldn't. She started to cry, but knew now was not the time. So she used her teeth to pull Tommy's blindfold off, then the gag. Once both were off, she listened to his breathing, calling his name as she nudged him with her shoulder.

Tommy had been lost in a state of suspended animation when he started to feel the pain return. He heard Helen's voice and opened his swollen eyes. Several hours must have passed, as the summer sun was no longer soft, but directly overhead, warm and harsh. He looked at Helen and smiled. After they were free, Helen attempted to clean Tommy, as she dressed him and then herself.

At home, their mother called the cops. Both children were rushed by EMS to a Queens Hospital.

"Tommy," Helen whispered to him as he lay in the hospital bed. "We promised, not to tell if they let us live."

"I had my fingers crossed, so it didn't count," he said with a grin.

"So did I," Helen said, as she tenderly hugged her defender, her friend, her little, big brother.

Willie was arrested, stood trial, but was never convicted. It was a waste of time and resources.

The same day the kids were abused, their father was found dead, bludgeoned with a pipe in their back yard. It was listed as a murder/robbery since all his money was gone. The perp or perps were never found.

Bobby went on to become a small-time crook, working construction sites as well as the Brooklyn Navy Yard. Death claimed him when he was ejected from a van. It rolled over where the Cross Island meets the Whitestone Expressway in Queens, New York. He was twenty-three years old at the time of his death.

Willie steered clear of Bobby after the court appearance but was killed four years later in a South Jamaica, Queens housing project by a rival gang.

Helen went on to marry a white-collar worker and become the mother of two. Her husband called 911 in the hope of forcing her to seek professional help to some dark hidden secret she would not discuss with him. As he explained it, at night he would awaken to find his wife just staring at the curtains, lost in a world of her own. Was that her brother lurking in the shadows? Even now, so many years after the event, even with his death, she still wakes up at night and wonders. The moment she wakes up, even today, she sees a figure lurking by the curtains in their master bedroom. The why wasn't important, but she needed to know if it was him. She always thought it was but never told Tommy of the haunting feeling.

Sometimes the psychological trauma is not only to the victim, but also to the crews. They are subject to untold stresses and never look at people the same again. The "Dance of Life" the crews perform is sometimes not as important to others as the patient's jewelry or wallet.

The patrol boss had been cruising around Northern Harlem, when he came down Edgecombe Avenue around 160th Street. It was a warm evening. The crew's compartment, once again, had no air conditioning working. But as far as the EMS civilian gods were concerned, that was okay. The crews could complain all they wanted; their complaints fell on deaf ears. But if the patient compartment did not have air conditioning, the bus was out of service.

There was a steady stream of jobs, creating another fast-moving evening for Nicola Halsey and me aboard Stress Free One Oh Zee. A continuous chatter emitted from our radio as jobs were being given out and acknowledged. The north frequency was never quiet. We sat on a corner, trying to catch a breeze, any breeze, awaiting our next assignment. People walked the streets. Children played next to dealers selling their trips to ecstasy.

Suddenly a patrol boss screamed, "Ten-thirteen! Ten-thirteen! I'm being dragged out of my vehicle."

Everyone, all the units on the frequency, tried to get a fix on him. We heard "Edgecombe," then we lost him.

"One Oh Zee. Heard, Edgecombe. Edgecombe. We're moving," Nickie yelled into the radio. In an unfashionable British manner, she had the pedal to the metal and we were ballistic. It would have made any Top Gun American fighter pilot proud, as we dodged traffic, heading toward Edgecombe.

Edgecombe and Macombs Place were two locations that had always been trouble spots. Thus there was a foreboding as we picked up Edgecombe up 155th Street. We started to shoot up the street. As we followed its lazy, curving form climbing northward, I looked to my right at the lush trees and green foliage lining the east side of the street.

This was the beginning of Highbridge Park. To the west, drab concrete monuments to man rose skyward. The beauty and splendor of Mother Nature beat man every time. It was only after we climbed the crest coming out of a slight curve that I spotted the lights of the command car, its door swung open with no supervisor in sight.

"Stress Free Double eight, on scene, Location Edgecombe and One Sixtieth Street," I said again, "Edgecombe, One Sixtieth Street. Need backup and PD forthwith. Crowd control."

I knew, by the size of the crowd, we were now in for trouble and wanted backup as fast as possible. In situations like this, we wanted a massive show of force, get our patient(s), and get out of the area. This means working on the patient after we are safely clear of the unrest. But this was one of our own and we had to find him.

Screw everyone else. Nickie and I bailed out to find the terrified, distraught patrol boss on his knees, pretending to be bagging a dead person. The patrol boss looked up with an agonizing, fearful look, as the people standing around him told him to "Do your job."

He was fumbling with the Bag Valve Mask, spraying himself with blood, as he knelt by the dead person.

The black male had brains coming out of his mouth and the crowd of blacks was increasing. As more arrived, they acted like uncontrolled, wild animals. The Basic unit of EMTs managed to get their bus closer to the scene.

"What do you need? Want a long board?" the EMT asked.

"Fuck that. Get us a stretcher fast," I yelled.

He realized what was happening, as people shoved and pushed us.

"Do something."

"Get him to the hospital."

"They don't care about no nigger."

Where the fuck are the cops? I thought. This was another case where the EMTs were literally saving the medics. They got a stretcher and we unceremoniously threw the body on it and ran. His brains and blood were splattering onto the dark asphalt street, turning it crimson red. The once white, crisp stretcher sheet was a bright red. We moved rapidly through the crowd. The perspiration poured off me. My dark green pants were soaked through in sweat.

Once in the back of the bus, I told the EMTs, "Let's get the fuck out of Dodge!"

I did not have to say it twice. The patrol boss was locked safely in his vehicle with a panicked look on his face. He ran to it as the irate crowd followed us. Nickie was at the dead guy's head, pretending to bag him with a blood- and brain-covered Bag Valve Mask. Each time she compressed the bag, blood shot out from his right ear.

I attempted to close the back doors. The crowd was rocking the bus, trying to turn us over. People climbed on top of each other to get through the back door. This was unreal. I caught sight of the EMT, as he looked through the hole from the crew to patient's compartment. He made it. Nickie yelled at him to get us out of here.

One clown got in, screaming, "I'm his brother. I want his gold."

Nickie recoiled in horror, as I knocked him out the back and managed to close one door.

"Let's get the fuck out of here," I kept saying. As I pulled on the second door, the vehicle was rocking from side to side. I looked at Nickie and saw real fear in her beautiful eyes. The crowd pulled, then screamed as I felt the vehicle lunge forward. The EMT was starting to move slowly, picking up speed. He was letting them know he did not give a shit who he ran down. The crowd was in a frenzy trying to get through the door. This overweight beast was trying to get in as I was pulling on the door.

"I'm his mother, you bastard. I want his gold."

She got a boot to the face and went tumbling out, taking several family members with her.

One hero was still hanging on to the rear light bar. He pulled up both feet and was about to kick me with his heavy construction boots. The clown must have watched a lot of videos. I nailed him in the balls and he went flying off the moving bus. I closed the door and sat down. I looked at this guy's body, then reached over, taking the remains of a slice of pizza covered in blood and brains that was stuck in his leather jacket. He was wearing a lot of gold.

"Hungry yet?" I asked Nickie, who was seated in the captain's chair. Blood was all over her white shirt. She was still holding the BVM and slumped back, looking exhausted.

A short time later, we pulled into Harlem Hospital with a dead person in the bus. As we took him out, we saw the damn crowd climbing out of cars. We ran into the crash room. The doctors and nurses moseyed on over in usual Harlem Hospital tradition. "What have you got?" asked a doctor.

"A dead person," I responded.

"Why did you bring him here?"

"For our safety. And by the way, doctor, you had better get the Hop Cops (Hospital Police) and PD here fast."

He only got to "Why . . ." when the door flung open and several people came screaming in, lunging for the body with its gold rings and only God knows how many chains. The EMTs, Nickie, and I realized the better part of valor was to leave the area. We headed out a side door, figuring after washing up, the riot would be under control enough to get a signature on our ACR for a dead person.

Soon the emergency bay, as well as the street that led to it, was awash in flashing red and white lights from the police cars. Much later that night, we talked to the patrol boss. He had been driving down Edgecombe when this individual went by him on his Ninja motorcycle. He was doing a wheelie. Up on the rear wheel with his helmet propped on the back of his head, he was eating a slice of pizza for all to see. Unfortunately, he didn't see the old oak tree that jumped out in front of him. There's a lesson to be learned here about the art of eating ethnic food. The patrol boss stopped and the crowd who had been watching him came upon the boss like flies on . . . Well, you get the picture.

FIVE

Just Another Day in Paradise

Here in the old EMS we worked hard, and we also played a lot of practical jokes. This one, however, didn't sit too well with the Mary Immaculate Unit it was played on.

It was on a hot, humid summer's evening in South Jamaica, Queens as a paramedic unit from a voluntary hospital responded to a "Shot."

They responded to find a crowd around a black male in his twenties who was lying unconscious in a pool of bright red blood. The crew grabbed their gear and started to work him in the street, as they requested a backup. The patient was the victim of a drive-by shooting. He was shot in the right leg, entry, no exit, and in his stomach, entry, no exit. A third round hit in his upper chest, entry, no exit.

As the crew feverishly worked, the mood of the crowd changed from tolerable and somewhat helpful, to menacing. The medic couldn't understand these people. They were trying to save a life, yet the crowd was increasingly hostile. After starting the two IVs, he looked up and saw what was motivating the fury. Through the rising steam of the boiling asphalt, he saw a black Rastafarian doll with dread locks hung on the front of their bus! A rope was around its neck, with several syringes stuck in the body!

Suddenly, not only the asphalt was heating up as tempers in the crowd rose.

"Holy shit," uttered one medic.

"Yeah, I know. The boy is fucked," said the other, after intubating him.

"Holy shit," reiterated the first medic, realizing someone was getting back at the wise-ass crew. The other medic looked up to see his petrified partner staring at the front of the bus.

"What?" he asked, turning, suddenly realizing they had been had.

"Holy fuckin' shit! Let's get the fuck out of here now."

They grabbed the patient on the long board, ran to the back of the bus, and threw in the equipment. People at the back hadn't seen the front. They helped lift the patient and were pleased at the speed of the two white medics.

"Is he getting worse?" asked a young woman in the crowd.

"Yeah," yelled the medic, "and it's going to get much worse if we don't get out of here now," he said, looking at his partner climbing into the driver's seat.

The crew cleared the scene in no time, amid a chorus of bottles and bricks ricocheting off the bus.

They took the patient to Mary Immaculate Hospital, better known as Mary Inaccurate, for obvious reasons. At the hospital, the doctor started to remove the occlusive dressing from the wound to the man's upper left chest and found chewing gum in the wound.

"What the hell?" the confused doctor said.

"Gee, maybe he was chewing gum and decided to use it as an occlusive dressing before we got there," the medic said. His partner, as well as the doctors, just looked at him. Outside, one medic was hysterical about how close they'd come to being killed.

"You have to chill out, man. You're just too sensitive for this job. Here, want a piece of chewing gum?" he said, reaching in and producing the pack.

"No fuckin' gum. No fuckin' backfiring. And no, I'm not working with you again!" He walked into the garage, signed in his drugs, and went home early.

Simeon Klebner and I pulled up to the Bagel Shop at Ninety-sixth Street and Broadway on the way up to the "Special Event." We supplied ourselves with "munchies" and started uptown. At 125th Street, we turned. The vehicle traffic was heavy, as crowds of people shopped at various stores. We came to a standstill approaching Lenox Avenue. About a hundred feet to our front was an EMS patrol vehicle.

"Let me get out and see what's happening," I said to Simeon, who was driving. As I started to get out, I heard several shots fired. Okay. No big deal. Shots were always going off in Harlem, as well as East New York. I could stand at the ambulance bay at Harlem Hospital on New Year's Eve and hear firepower that would make any infantry veteran proud.

I went out into the crowd. They too heard the shots, but if it wasn't cracking across your ear, no big deal. A patrol boss from Staten Island got on the PA and screamed, "Shots fired, run!"

I dove back into the bus, as a once calm sea of black humanity became an instant tidal wave of insanity storming the vehicle. People right up the front of the vehicle, climbing on the patient compartment and jumping off behind, onto the street! Some made pretty lousy falls and lay there screaming for help.

"Let's get the fuck out of here," I yelled to Sim.

"What about the boss?"

"Fuck that asshole. Let's get to the MERV."

We took a right and moved out with lights, the siren wailing, not stopping for anyone. We headed toward the MERV, two blocks away. People begged us for help.

We yelled, "The ambulance behind us will help." Of course there was no one behind us, but we had to get to the MERV. Once we arrived, I hoped someone would have the brains to marshal the EMS resources and develop a plan to help the people. But from the screams over our radio, I knew things were chaotic.

People stormed the MERV, trying to hold onto the officer and gain access to the MERV. One of the EMTs pulled a lieutenant to safety into the MERV by his belt. The crew fought to secure the door and hatches. The area around the vehicle was a war zone, totally devastated. The surging black storm overturned tables, chairs, and lives. The panicked mob approached the other units parked by the MERV. One crew couldn't get into their vehicle. They leapt under its giant rear axles, screaming "Ten-thirteen! Ten-thirteen!" into their portable as shots continued to ring out.

The crest of humanity overran, then moved beyond, the MERV. A loudmouth black captain told a white EMT, "Get your ass out of your vehicle and go into that crowd and see who's hurt."

"Fuck you," responded the EMT. "I'll follow you."

Needless to say, no one went. Cops poured into the area and the shooting started to die down. The collateral damage from the havoc instigated by the idiot patrol boss was extensive. People had crush injuries from being trampled, heart attacks, and broken bones from being struck by flying material. We had several patients who were burned with hot oil as the rampaging crowds overturned stoves. All of this was because of one idiot's mouth.

Arty Gonzales is better known as "10-62-02" (out of service and in need of oxygen) by crew members who feel he is less than competent at picking up his share of jobs. I like him.

Sitting on Forty-second Street about seventy-five feet from Third Avenue, we observed a young girl fly by on roller blades, at a high rate of speed. Arty was concerned, "I don't think she is going to stop." His heart is in the right place, though at times judgment may be muddied.

He realized if she didn't, she would be struck by the faster-moving traffic, jetting north on Third Avenue.

"She'll stop," I said, in an almost bored tone. *Crash! Bam! Pow!* "Told you she'd stop," I said, looking at him. She came to an ungraceful halt by slamming into the back of a small hatchback, having approached the vehicle at a high rate of speed and bodyslamming it. The impact sounded like the collision of two trucks.

When I got to her, she was sitting on the ground. A pedestrian helped me remove a leather jacket, as another held head stabilization to ensure her head wouldn't move. Arty brought up a long board. These civilians were great! Too often we never get the chance to thank them.

She was bleeding from the mouth, had a gash on her face, and complained of chest pain. A crowd had formed and I heard Lieutenant Paul Giblin, Navy Seal, on the scene.

We got her strapped to the board, when I heard someone ask which hospital she'd go to.

"She'll go to Bellevue," Arty said. "She have bwain matter coming out her mouth." I did a double take and looked at the patient. "Bwain matter?" Well he does have a way with words. I tried not to laugh. After we got her into the back of the bus, I closed the door on everyone. As she lay there, I reached over and removed the gray gum, *brain matter*, Arty was talking about. As I examined her, I lectured the kid, who was about fourteen years old, on high-speed roller blades with no helmets. After checking her, I asked why she continued to cry.

Looking at me with doe-like eyes, she said, "I'm a model. My life is over."

She had me open her book bag and pull out a portfolio. She was a model from Brazil, working with an agency. We got her to Bellevue. Her mother and aunt arrived and both were cool, gracious, people. They had plans of warming her butt once she got back to Rio to get plastic surgery. I wasn't sure where the plastic surgery would be needed more.

A crew got called for a distraught citizen. The guy had been walking down the street and spotted a Knicks jacket on the ground. Figuring he found a bargain, our hapless citizen snatched it up. From within, something rolled out. No, it wasn't a basketball. It was a head, professionally chopped off. The victim, a light-skinned black, had duct tape across his mouth. His opened eyes showed a hurt look.

After a head is cut off, there is oxygen in the brain for a good four to six minutes. With your head separated from the body, you are still alive.

The unit took pictures. Several days later, a photo of the head was found in the garage with the name of an old song pasted below it, "I Ain't Got No Body."

It was a beautiful autumn day in the Big Apple and I had the pleasure of working with paramedic Byron Melo, nicknamed the "Colombian Navy Seal." I couldn't help but have an enjoyable day when I worked with this gentleman. His humor was really cutting.

Saturday mornings in Manhattan were a special treat. The only ones out and about were us and tourists. Once in a while a sector would pass, but even the terrorist yellow cabs had not unleashed their fury on the city yet. The air was fresh and clean as we drove past the Empire State Building. After coffee, we sat at Thirty-fourth Street and Madison Avenue and checked out the gems at the Astro Gallery. We moved up to Fifth Avenue and sipped our coffee, as we watched the tourists flock to the building King Kong climbed.

The FM played soft oldies and the smell of fresh roasted peanuts lingered in the air. Across the street, a tourist bus emptied its load of Japanese schoolgirls as a German couple took pictures. A gaily dressed African woman window-shopped.

The call came for an "Unconscious." We'd go alone until we confirmed the job. This was the latest in stupidity from the fire gods. On subway jobs, where our radios don't work, we were sent alone. The genius in communication called it utilization of resources. Since we were understaffed, management wanted to keep a bus available for another call. Thus the patient suffered and the crews got ulcers.

We responded to Forty-second Street and Park Avenue. On a bus was our "Unconscious," which was an "Arrest."

The bus was smaller than a city mass-transit bus. The gentleman, a black male in his early fifties, was traveling with his wife. He had a history of hypertension. He developed chest pains. And slumped in a tight seat next to his wife.

Byron grabbed him from behind to place him on the floor, but he was massive. I got behind him and had to gorilla him to the floor, wrenching my back. The call was in for a backup. The Dance of Life began. Byron started bagging the patient until I could get him the intubation set. I did CPR and hooked him to the cardiac monitor.

He had that flat rhythm we will all go into. I passed the intubation set to Byron. He was much smaller than me and he was able to get a better position to do the intubation.

An engine pulled up. "What can we do? Do you want him put on your stretcher?"

"No. We need one of your guys to do CPR," I told the fire captain.

"You got it and anything else you need."

There were engines with firemen and officers who did the right thing. Engine One, Ladder Seven, Engine Sixteen, Rescue One, had always been supportive and professional. These guys reflected how the system was supposed to work. But they were not the majority.

Unlike these units, 99.9 percent of the engine crews did not get off their trucks, if they even got to the job. In Manhattan they'd be assigned, then canceled with an "Unable to validate address." This usually happened on subway jobs. Bet your sweet ass they could validate the address if there was a fire or cameraman. Considering they spent fewer than four hours on the street every twenty-four hours, perhaps some time should have been spent in map reading classes.

The wife sat there as I was bent over the seat, pushing medication, trying to get just one cell to explode with life. One fireman hung over a seat, doing good compressions. Byron was on the floor, attempting to get the patient tubed. We both realized if we didn't get him here, in the bus, they would never get him back at the hospital. After the first round of medications, we got the spark of hope as the monitor came to life and we felt pulses.

I decided to move to Bellevue Hospital, bus and all. We gave notification to Bellevue, asking for extra hands. We traveled in a convoy of a car, a fire engine, and the bus with us on board, followed by a Basic unit from Cabrini Hospital. One EMT drove their ambulance, while the other drove ours. Lights and sirens wailed as we bounced on the floor and lost, then got back, the patient's pulse. I pushed more medications and Byron bagged him.

Several minutes later, the five-vehicle convoy turned into the Bellevue Hospital grounds. The bus was directed to pull into the emergency ambulance bay as we lost him again.

As the door opened, I tried to stand. My back was killing me, when a third-year doctor bolted onto the bus.

"Let's do some real CPR," he proclaimed in front of a shocked wife.

I looked at the sweat-covered fireman who was doing good CPR and said, "Continue." Then I turned, "You," talking to the doctor, "get off the bus, now!" EMT Konstantinos "Gus" Scamalos, a burly, good-natured Greek, "assisted" Ben Casey off the bus. The old adage was true, "Paramedics save patients, but EMTs save the paramedics."

Dr. William Goldberg, wearing a business suit, climbed on board. I gave him a fast SITRAP (Situation Report). Byron had not been able to get the tube in, although we got pulses back. Dr. Goldberg, one of Bellevue Hospital's best, climbed over the seats, took off his jacket, and wiggled between seats onto the bus floor.

As a fireman and I pulled up the patient, Byron provided cricoid pressure. (This is pressure to a specific portion of the throat, which allows the person doing the intubation to visualize the target better.) Dr. Goldberg got a successful intubation.

We decided to move the patient. EMTs Scamalos, Deirdre Fahy, Ashley Alejo, Karl Dykman, and Reggie Jenkins pushed past the hospital staff to remove the patient with the assistance of the firemen. I couldn't help but love these EMS people. Once the patient was on the hospital stretcher, his lung sounds were checked to make sure the tube had not moved, and he was whisked into the emergency room. His wife, even in her grief and state of shock, was gracious to us. I apologized to the fireman for the stupid remark by the brainless third-year doctor. Within a few minutes, an EMS supervisor ordered the units to get to their street locations.

The call came in as a "Cardiac" so we responded. The sky was crystal clear and the breeze crisp, as the 10Z pulled in front of the dreary red apartment building. As we unloaded the cardiac monitor, heavy drug bag, portable oxygen bottle in bag, and stair chair, we each remarked about the pearl-like features of the full autumn moon. Its light and the beautiful stars glittering above energized a tired crew.

Upstairs, we entered a clean apartment. The patient's husband answered the door. He was a thin, boring-type guy who led us into the kitchen. Even the lighting in the kitchen, though providing ample visibility, did nothing to liven up the apartment's depressed atmosphere. It was as if we had stepped into a time warp: "The World of the Monotonous and Uninteresting."

A woman in her early fifties sat at the kitchen table. She was dressed in a pastel blouse with dark brown pants. A lackluster gray bun sat at the back of her head, held by large bobby pins. Her shoulders were hunched and hands loosely clasped on the table in front of her.

After I dropped the fifty pounds of equipment, I checked for a pulse, first mine then the patient's. My partner Harvey and I had entered another dimension and both felt our own energy drained by the environment, the husband, and the patient.

"How can we help you, ma'am?" I asked, trying not to laugh as Harvey kept checking his pulse in an overexaggerating manner.

"Oh, I have this pain here," she said in a monotonous voice.

"Okay. What were you doing when the pain developed?"

"I was trying to close the window."

She had pulled her shoulder muscle closing the living room window. After we finished our evaluation and were satisfied it was a muscular problem, we asked if she wanted to go to the hospital.

"How long will I have to wait?" she asked in a lifeless tone that would make you think about killing yourself for some excitement.

"Probably several hours, at least."

"What will they give me?"

God, even the plants by the windows were dying! Talk about a depleted energy field!

"Probably some Motrin," I said.

"And a fantastic bill for the emergency room visit and doctor's consult," Harvey chimed in, observing me getting as depressed as she was.

"Thanks," I said.

"Oh, oh, what can I do?"

"Well, first, if you don't want to go to the hospital, you need to sign this form releasing us." In an agonizingly slow pace, she put on her dull gray-framed glasses and started to sign the form.

When she finished her herculean task of signing her name, she asked, "And what else?"

"Well you could get some massage oil . . ."

But before I could finish, she whiningly said, "But I don't have any massage oil."

"Okay. Well, do you have any Bertolli Extra Virgin Imported Olive Oil?"

"Yes."

"Okay, then have your husband massage your shoulder and don't sleep by an open window tonight."

"But I want you to massage me, not him."

"Uh, ma'am, although I went to school for massage therapy, I'm here in an emergency capacity," I said, standing up.

"But you are supposed to help people."

"Yes, we can take you to the hospital."

"They won't heal me like you will. Donald, get the olive oil now!"

The husband got the oil and a towel. I looked at Harvey and sheepishly smiled. Healing is in the mind of the patient, no matter what the modality. Without missing a beat, Harvey picked up the radio and gave the dispatcher an "Extended on the scene, patient care."

"Well, I can't massage you with your blouse on. I need to see your shoulder." She moved as fast as the Iraqi Army surrendering! Like a rocket she ran into the bedroom, returning in a housecoat.

"Where do you want *to do me*? The bedroom?" she anxiously asked in a deeply sensual voice.

Harvey made a gesture with his eyebrows. Turning to the patient, I said, "Oh no. *I'll do you* right there in the living room on the couch where *everyone* can watch."

Kinky is as kinky does. She moved to the couch, opening the housecoat slowly, allowing it to now only partially cover her pronounced naked backside, which was clearly visible.

"I'm ready," she purred like a child receiving a birthday gift.

I smiled as the husband stood holding the towel. After heating the oil on the stove, I started to warm the patient with a massage. As I worked her shoulder and back, she started to moan. I looked at Harvey, who was now making eyes showing surprise that I was actually getting such a reaction.

"Please do me," she pleaded, squirming. "It feels so good . . . more."

"Sorry, that's the shoulder, arm, and adjoining back. That's all."

"Please. This is fantastic." The housecoat slid further down her legs.

"Yes, it is, and I'm sure Donald can finish the rest."

"But I want you," now sounding like a jilted child.

"Sorry. It does feel better, doesn't it?"

"Oh, yes!"

"Good, then Donald can finish you. Goodnight."

I took the towel from the husband, washed in the kitchen sink, grabbed the equipment and we left the now practically naked and frustrated patient on the couch. Dull Donald stood silently in the living room, towel draped on his arm where I placed it, still holding the cup of oil in his hand.

In the hallway, Harvey kept staring at me. Finally smiling, "Out of more than eight million people in this city, you get the one who asks for a massage. Amazing!"

Yes, we paramedics are multi-talented. As paramedics, we realize, more than doctors, that medicine is an art and not a science. Some of us are just more artistic than most.

It had been a long day aboard 19 Victor in the heart of the South Bronx. My partner, paramedic Mark Taylor, and I were working overtime. We were called for a "Cardiac/Respiratory Arrest." The location was a lot at West 170 and Cromwell Avenue.

We turned the corner and saw the lights of the Basic unit, 17 Henry, and Engine 42 proclaiming our arrival. The red and white flashing lights harshly broke the beauty of the picturesque purple sky at dusk. We grabbed our gear and started our ascent over the dilapidated remnants of a cinder block wall. We climbed upward through the forbidding hill of weeds and garbage alongside a building. At the crest was a clear area where the patient lay on the soft earth. The crew of 17 Henry, EMTs J. Moritz and M. Daddona from Battalion Fifty-five, had already moved the young female out of her filthy shanty. It was located on the side of the hill about one hundred and fifty feet from where we entered and a good fifty feet above the street. Along with the firemen from Engine Forty-two, they stripped her and started the Dance for Life.

It was getting dark as my partner lay on the ground and tubed her. With no IV access in her arms or neck, I lay at her feet in the dirt and filth, finally getting a line in the top of her foot. Her junkie friends lashed out at the patient, Edna, and then at us, for our inability to save her. The squalor was unbelievable. The patient evidently had overdosed on methadone.

She lay looking at the full moon peacefully entering the rich velvet sky. Her young, brown body, scarred by years of shooting drugs, lay lifeless in the dust and filth.

Strangers performed a Dance of Life around her. How sad, her friends cursed her while EMTs, paramedics, and firemen fought for one of the dregs of society. In their hearts, these strangers believed this junkie's life was worth their time, effort, and talent. They joined together on this filthy, barren hill in the South Bronx and fought the Grim Reaper. When everyone else abandoned her, when her friends cursed her, when she no longer believed in her own self-worth, these Street Saints of Compassion believed she was priceless.

I knew she was gone. She was gone long before we got there. Her trip into another dimension had begun and I prayed she had learned all her lessons. After expending our life-saving medications with no change from that basic rhythm we all know, asystole, flat line, it was over. My partner journeyed down the hill to call for termination. In this moment of silence, I felt a precious energy of peace and love. Across eternity, I knew Edna was happy with us all.

Mark called telemetry and talked with a Dr. White. When the doctor learned she was thirty-four, he went ballistic and wanted her transported to a hospital. He didn't have a clue, nor would he accept the fact she was dead as a doornail. I accepted it as a typical remark from a non–street-smart doctor and a mockery of paramedicine. Our unit transported her to Bronx Lebanon Hospital, the closest. The staff saw us bring in an arrest with the EMTs doing compressions, and so on. Before we could say anything, the nurse asked, "How old?"

"Thirty-four."

"Are you sure? She looks young and should be in Pediatrics."

"Look! She's—" Before I could finish, a doctor asked, "What are her vital signs?"

"Okay! That's it. Everybody stop!" I yelled to the two stunned EMTs. Not from my yelling but the total stupidity from the rocket scientists of Bronx Lebanon Hospital.

"This is an arrest! An adult dead patient! Dead as throw dirt on you and not let you out on weekends! Dead as there are no vital signs from her just like your fuckin' brain-dead staff!" The doctor called the code. Outside we had some unkind remarks about our EMS Dr. White.

Medicine is an art, not science. The same is true of predicting the weather. Being artistic paramedics, we developed a method to predict tomorrow's weather. Instruments? Hell with the crap cardiac monitors we were given, we developed our system with observation only.

Paramedic Tom Reynolds and I were sitting by Seventy-second Street and Broadway, checking out the girls. It was one of those priceless, warm summer nights when I asked myself, "Shouldn't I be in Barbados? Or even Bosnia? Not sitting in a bus without air conditioning in the crew compartment. Why the hell are we sucking in diesel fumes, known to cause cancer and respiratory and cardiac diseases?

Diesel fuel contains more than forty cancer-causing agents. It also creates cardiac and asthma problems, to say nothing about killing the environment.

Tom and I laughed at the prediction, "No rain for tonight and tomorrow." We developed a surefire method for detecting rain, way in advance. It is based on a paramedic study. We sat in the bus and checked out the glorious, bra-less breasts and did not detect one nipple erection. Prior to rain, the electrical field in the atmosphere changed. This shift in electrons created nipple erections, creating an early warning system for a change in the weather. We might not get the Nobel prize for science, but we put in long hours conducting our study.

Suzie "I'm a nurse" came up, telling us we were needed, and left. Would you expect less from a nurse? We pulled up to find one of the local drunks on the sidewalk. I got out and walked over. I gingerly kicked his foot and he sat up.

In the middle of Yuppieville, this homeless drunk lay in his own shit with flies congregating on him. He was shoeless and his pants showed clearly where his urine and feces had gone. He had lice in his hair, needed a shave, and held a quart bottle of beer in his filthy, feces-covered hand.

"Okay, pop. You can't stay here," I said, realizing there was no way in hell he was going anywhere unless we took him.

"We are going to take you to the hospital." Something caught my eye, so I put on some gloves and pulled up his pant leg. From his ankle to knee, he was a mass of white maggots.

"Fuck us," I said, as Tom shook his head.

"I'll get the kit," he said.

The kit included a paper-thin gown, gloves, and mask with eye protector. As I was donning mine, two Yuppies stopped and looked.

"Take a walk," Tommy told them.

They stood and gawked.

"Hey, he needs a home," I said, as I went to grab their hands.

"Come on. If you are so interested, help."

The two losers ran off, briefcases swinging in the wind. As I tied the gown behind my back, a Mexican flower vendor approached. Without saying a word, he reached behind me and tied the gown.

"Gracias, amigo," I said.

He smiled and walked away.

"I'm not going to no hospital if I can't finish my beer," our belligerent drunk said.

"Hey, no problem. I give you my word that after we get you into the back of the bus I'll give it to you."

"Are you sure?" he asked warily.

"Trust me," I knelt down and wrapped his maggot-covered leg with two red plastic bags, then taped them to his leg. Next we double-wrapped the sheets on the stretcher with a blanket at the base. We loaded him and his thousands of friends running up our arms. I climbed in the back and before he could say anything, I gave him his beer.

"You did keep your word," he said with a smile.

"I told you to trust me. Now give me your arm."

Tommy looked, "What are you doing?"

"Getting the vitals and checking him out, that's what." Tom shook his head. I reached over and set up a non-rebreather oxygen mask.

"Oh, I don't need no oxygen," he said, taking another drink of his Colt beer.

"You don't, but I sure do." His aroma was so overpowering I put the oxygen on myself. Tom completed the ACR and handed it to me. For a moment he looked at me.

"What?" I asked.

"This is another one of those EMS paramedic moments. Him drinking his beer and you with the oxygen mask on."

We finally pulled into Roosevelt, closest hospital. I opened the back door and dumped the empty beer bottle and took off my oxygen mask. Tom and I lifted out the patient and rolled him in.

Roosevelt is known for its less-than-amiable nurses. One in particular was a middle-aged, plump blonde and anything but a nice person. Her buddy looked like an emaciated witch. Her distended, hooked nose, black hair, and squeaky voice underscored her total lack of human personality.

As we rolled the patient into the emergency room, his odor preceded us. I rolled him over to the triage area. The registrar got up and moved out. Miss Blonde looked at me with fire in her eyes

"Why didn't you take it to Bellevue or Saint Clare's Hospitals?" she sarcastically asked. I looked at her as the doctors headed for the doors. No one approached the patient.

"This is a patient," I yelled. "I can't feel the love," I screamed louder. "Where is the love?"

Needless to say, they wanted me out of there. They begrudgingly took our patient.

After Roosevelt Hospital got rid of the 911 paramedic and EMT units, their receiving in the emergency room dropped through the floor. It got so bad, EMS units were pressured to bring patients to the hospital. EMS chiefs sent out the gestapo, BITS (Bureau of Investigation and Trials), as well as EMS supervisors to pressure and intimidate units to take patients to Roosevelt Hospital because it was the closest, but not necessarily the best.

It's a shame the doctor who headed the ER never had a clue as to the problem. It sure as hell was not the EMS crews. Finally, they had to bring back and run ambulances from the hospital. This would ensure patients went to *their hospital*. Is this steering or am I missing something?

Prior to this episode, we had picked up a black Jamaican female, who had SVT (supraventricular tachycardia); her heart was going crazy and beating too fast.

When we asked her where she wanted to go, she said Roosevelt. She sensed my hesitation as I said she'd soon find out why for herself. I knew the witch was on duty.

The witch came over and started treating the woman like crap. It didn't take long before the woman started yelling at the nurse. She was accustomed to being treated as a black, but she let it be known she was a prominent professor. When the witch realized whom she was dealing with, her whole demeanor changed.

As I walked out the door, the professor called to me, "Thanks, Jim. Now I know what you meant." I smiled. Justice is sweet.

I hadn't seen the witch in a good Halloween. Perhaps, she flew somewhere else. For the sake of the hospital and patients, I sure hope so.

The lesson here was one the doctors often missed. It was the nurses who made an Emergency Room. The hospital administrator ran to the civilian gods of EMS and threatened their egos. But in the end, the problems were due to ineptness by the nurses. If they checked Beth Israel's staff of nurses they would learn what being an emergency room nurse meant.

So you think date rape only happens to little foolish girls? Think again, this is New York City.

The EMTs were on the scene calling for medic backup. Tommy and I responded, not sure what we would find since the situation report wasn't clear.

Once there we loaded our gear and headed into the tenement. The building was dark and dreary. *How strange,* I thought, as Tom cursed at the strain of carrying the ungainly cardiac monitor on the almost vertical ascent. A male's voice called out, "They're in here."

Their landing was small. A white male, about twenty, held open the door. He stood about five feet three inches and wore only black pants. His narrow, pasty face sported a slight, black goatee. Silver glittered from his pierced ears, nose, and navel. Small chains of silver hung from his nipples.

As we stepped in, I noticed rings on his toes and a six-foot glass case to the left. As our eyes adjusted to the dim light, we could see a large python snake.

"My friend needs help," he said in a squeaky voice.

"What's your friend's name?" I asked, as we were directed into the living room.

"I don't know. I just met him."

As we entered, there were two EMTs attempting to pull a male's shorts and pants up from his ankles. The arched, twelve-foot window illuminated the messy, sparsely furnished room.

The two EMTs tried to pull up the male's shorts and pants, but he was being combative.

"Okay, roll him over," I said. Tommy and I noticed the man's pupils were mere pinpoints and his respirations were decreasing. Then two officers walked in.

"Okay. So what did you give him?" I asked the "new friend" as Tom drew up the Narcan.

"Nothing! I have no idea of what you are talking about."

I looked at the cops then back at the male.

"Yeah, right. Do you need us?" the cops asked, realizing what had taken place and not wanting to make a collar even if the patient made the complaint.

"Nah, you can go. Have a safe tour."

"You too," they said with a sigh of relief.

"You don't have to be so nasty," the male said in a voice only a mother could love because the father would kill him. He now was posturing with his arms crossed, tapping his foot on the worn rug directly in front of me. "I'm talking to you!" His tone got higher as I ignored him and gave the patient the Narcan. The two new EMTs were in a total state of confusion, not knowing what to do, trying to use a BVM on the floundering patient.

"Hey you! I'm talking to you."

Tommy smiled.

"I think the, uh, gentleman likes you," he said with a typical Tommy smirk.

"Hey," the guy yelled.

I had enough, "Listen, Tinkerbell . . ."

"What? What did you call me?"

Tommy broke up laughing.

"I want your name and shield. How . . ."

Before he could finish his statement, I yelled, "Hey!"

At that moment the Narcan had kicked in and the patient said, "What?"

Tommy and I laughed and the two new EMTs snickered.

"Not you," I said. "You! Tinkerbell. Open your fuckin' mouth again I'll call back the cops and have your ass arrested. We all know what happened here."

The man's eyes glared at me.

"I'm sure the boys in central booking and department of corrections will enjoy a little fudge package like you. See how much you enjoy taking it up the ass all day."

"He'd probably enjoy it a lot. Make a good prison bitch," remarked Tom, smiling. "Hey, whatever you enjoy is fine with me. But knocking someone out is rape."

With this the male shut up.

"Okay, let's package up the love child," I said to the two distraught EMTs. The patient was still a little groggy, but was able to stand and walk to the bus. In the back of the bus, the six-foot, blond Irish lad asked the EMT what happened.

"We found you on the floor with your pants and shorts down to your ankles. Your ass was in the air. Do you know the meaning of safe sex?"

The kid was starting to learn.

Date rape drugs made a big splash in the newspapers when they were used on girls. In Manhattan we picked up more guys than girls having had drugs used on them. At one of the gay clubs, it got to be such a regular occurrence that the EMTs no longer called for medics. They supported the patient's airway and took him to the hospital. EMTs do save paramedics.

One night, Jack Ng and I received an "Asthma" call. As we exited the vehicle, the people screamed at us to hurry, "She's turning black."

We entered the bedroom to find a young girl, semi-nude on a bed, unresponsive, and covered in vomit. She was in respiratory arrest. We lowered her to the floor.

Jack cleared as much of the vomit as he could before intubating her. I hooked her to the cardiac monitor, got an IV line, and gave her the first round of medications. As we worked, we were witnessing this kid's death. I called for backup, explaining it was a pediatric arrest.

Tara McEvoy, a great EMT from Station Eleven, and her partner responded. We continued the Dance of Life at an accelerated rate.

Fighting against hope, we packaged the kid. Tara gave an urgent notification to Beth Israel Hospital to stand by. It was the closest and second only to Bellevue in its care.

Jack and I fought for her life. Bouncing around in the back of the bus, we gave the child more medication as Tara swerved and struggled through the traffic. After a brief, hectic trip, we pulled into Beth Israel. The staff was waiting as we brought the child into the crash room. The staff at Beth Israel made a point of working with the crew. When we brought in the child, it was not a matter of dumping or even transferring her. It was a matter of assisting the patient to the next higher medical expert.

As the doctors and nurses took over the Dance of Life, I walked outside. Both Jack and I were soaked in sweat. I thanked Tara and her partner as I asked Jack for the child's name. I had Masses said for some of my patients, but especially for the kids.

"Celina," he said. It hit me like a rock as I told him her name, age, and address. Celina was a thirteen-year-old who grew up on the lower East Side of Manhattan. She was priority asthma, and I had responded to her call with different partners numerous times before, for she had been intubated too many times in her young life. All the crews fell in love with this special lady.

Walking inside as the code continued, I tapped a nurse who was giving CPR. I stepped up and placed my sweat-soaked hands on Celina's bare, cold chest and started compressions. As I worked, totally devastated, I functioned automatically as a professional NYC paramedic, talking to the doctor, giving the child's history.

Dr. Barbara went beyond the human touch and I will never forget her for it. She looked at me and said, "There's nothing more that can be done. Jim, do you want anything else done?" I will never forget this doctor's compassion. She was a healer, not just a doctor. I realized it was over and thanked her. I slowly walked outside as Jack was doing the paperwork, and he asked if I was all right. Then it hit him. He had often heard me talk of the child. He and I started to cry.

After a few minutes, I asked a nurse to walk with me. Entering the empty code room, I saw Celina under a white sheet. They had already extubated her. Under the stark lights, I gently pulled back the crisp, white sheet and looked. Her hair was in a bun. I wiped off some dried vomit from around her small, delicate mouth. Then, I bent over and kissed her. My tears fell onto her face, forming puddles in her lifeless, closed eyes. Slowly the tears overflowed and ran down her cheeks. I tenderly covered her and walked to the door, where the nurse stood.

"You never saw anything," I said. The nurse hugged me. I wiped the tears away from my eyes, walking out into the dark night. Jack joined me and I was glad he was my partner this night, but even more my friend.

As we pulled away from the hospital, we hit the available signal. A short time later, we were told to report to Station Eleven. We didn't notice the dispatcher had changed our signal to "Out of Service." Out of concern for our loss, Tara had spoken to Lieutenant Juan Torres. He took the initiative to put us off service. He wanted to know if I wanted to take the rest of the night off.

I said, "No. I have to stay available and get the tour completed."

He called Lieutenant "Pinkie" Alberme, better known as Lieutenant Albuterol, at Station Thirteen, Bellevue. They agreed we should take the following day off.

EMTs and paramedics do not have a "Heart Bill." We do not have health coverage should we have a heart attack. Yet when we treat patients, we pay dearly with our hearts.

I learned that Celina had argued with her mother and went to her uncle's apartment upset, with an asthma attack. She went into the bathroom and turned on the steam. The uncle forgot about her for thirty minutes. When he finally decided to check on her, he found the child unconscious. Instead of calling 911 and getting help, he carried her into a bedroom, stripped her to the waist, and started compressions on the bed. This was totally useless. Next, he blew into her mouth without hyperextending the child's head. Instead of air entering her lungs, it entered her stomach. Thus, she vomited. The vomit entered her lungs, burning and destroying them. These actions killed the child.

For several weeks, I was gun shy. I could understand an adult's passing better than a child's. Having lost my wife, my best friend, before our second year together, I did not accept death easily. If anything, I fought harder. With maturity of the spirit, I learned that no matter what age, everyone has an appointed time. Celina, as well as my Melanie, had lessons to learn and lessons to teach. Sometimes, the hardest lesson to learn is love.

Two weeks later, Jack and I were deployed to Harlem and received a "Pediatric Asthma." We raced through the Harlem streets, each driven by a traumatic urgency. We blasted through an intersection. As I cleared my side for oncoming traffic, I saw a young girl. She was in her mid-twenties, standing with friends. She turned, stepped away from the group, and faced us. I made eye contact for a split second. As I looked at her slender regal African features, she made the sign of the cross and held her hands out. With palms facing us, she lowered her head. I caught a view of her in the mirror as she returned to her fiends. Her act of love still brings tears to my eyes.

We pulled up to the old tenement. A young, black female about nineteen ran to us.

"Thank God you're here," she screamed. "My sister said she could hear you guys and needed you really bad."

"Where is she?" I asked.

"Inside. Please hurry!"

We entered the apartment and saw the twelve-year-old on the barren, wooden floor. Jack went for the pulse. She was dead. No pulse, no respirations. An older, black gentleman ushered the neighbors out of the way so we could work. I intubated her as Jack got the IV and monitor. At the same time, we instructed the sister on how to do compressions. There was no time to waste calling for a backup. We pushed medications and then pushed more. The cardiac monitor still showed asystole, flat line, death. Then it happened—our little Harlem miracle.

"Check for a pulse," I heard Jack say.

Sure enough, we had a pulse, a blood pressure, and a perfect rhythm. And then the little princess opened her beautiful, brown eyes. I spoke to her and she was able to follow commands. Her sister cried, hugging us both. The child, by the grace of God, had no brain damage and left Harlem Hospital the next afternoon. A lot can be accomplished with love.

Each day, the Street Saints of Compassion entered a world that few understood. As we entered our stations, we brought our immediate emotional baggage. Perhaps we had an argument with our wife, husband, or significant other. Perhaps a child was sick. As we approached our station, we wondered what crap would come across the desk at us, even before we began dealing with patients.

After we signed for our narcotics and radio, we checked out the unit. Many days we were not even at the unit when the supervisor notified the communication center we were available for jobs. He was worried about getting a unit into service, to keep the captain off his ass. The captain was in a fog, with visions of promotion to chief. The chief needed to generate paperwork to justify his existence and used intimidation to feel like a man.

At the unit, we checked out the equipment. If we did not stay on top of this, it would take forever. Often, the tour we relieved got in late and left the bus like a shit-house, smell included. Communications screamed they had jobs and needed us. When we explained we had not had the chance to check the bus, this overweight donut said in a belittling manner, "Are you refusing a job? If so, you are out of service."

Few supervisors would get on the radio and intercede for the unit. Because we didn't want charges, we would accept the job without checking the bus. We told the dispatcher we were responding. Next, we asked the dispatcher to document we were going unchecked, in case we were brought up on charges for missing equipment. It was rare to have a dispatcher acknowledge this request. Usually we heard, "All I need to hear is that you are responding." So the pressure increased.

As we pulled up to the scene we often saw the ELI, the little red fire truck up the block waiting for us. ELI stands for "Emergency Light Indicator," since that is what most of them are. They were not staying, surprise, or even getting off the truck, bigger no surprise. They pretended to have a "bad address." In reality, they waited for us to pull up so they could leave.

On the scene, the crew unloaded the drug bag, cardiac monitor, oxygen bag, and stair chair. Next, they climbed the five-floor walkup and found that the patient was having an AMI (acute myocardial infarct), a big-league heart attack. The patient was a sixty-year-old Polish gentleman who spoke no English. The Dance of Life began.

The crew worked feverishly to save his life. Once the basics were finished, physical assessment, blood pressure, pulse, lung sounds, oxygen on, IV access gained, first-round drugs delivered, they realized the patient had a problem. Instead of getting better, he was "circling the drain"—dying. They got on the phone to request morphine. The patient became more combative as he fought to live. Then they requested EMS Basic backup forthwith.

The dispatcher asked for a condition.

By now the crew were on adrenaline and one of them told him, "Imminent arrest. I want EMTs, not fire."

That statement would surely get them a lecture at the very least.

His partner was on the phone with a telemetry doctor. The doctor was annoyed at being bothered, as he had to put down his newspaper. Seems he lost money in the stock market. The medic explained the situation and the request. The doctor gave him orders completely out of protocol, as well as out of this world. Once again, the medic explained the patient to the doctor. This time, he stopped halfway through and said, "Doc, please explain this to my partner," and he handed me the phone.

Upon hearing the doctor, the medic was in shock, made an excuse and hung up.

Finally the backup came in, wearing bunker gear; they were firemen.

That fuckin' dispatcher, the medic thought.

Perhaps if you bastards got your asses off your fuckin' truck in the first place, we could be in our bus by now, he thought.

The Ring of Concern, firemen, prompted by the lieutenant, couldn't do enough for them. They realized they fucked up but did not want to be burned. They figured, be nice to EMS and the crew wouldn't say anything. Wisely, the partners opted to hold off on the doctor's order because it would have killed the patient. If he had any hope, it was for the crew to run to a qualified hospital. We knew the hospitals that saved lives.

After the heroes almost dropped the patient in the chair, the crew decided to carry him. Going down the stairs, they said a silent prayer that the Piss Patches (EMTs) would arrive. Downstairs, as they loaded the patient into the bus, the EMTs pulled up. The paramedics said a silent prayer of thanks since these Piss Patches were the best in the business.

Day in, day out, paramedics saved patients. But few paramedics would acknowledge their admiration for the EMTs who save paramedics. Later they would find out that the EMTs heard the call and buffed the job to bail them out. That means they weren't assigned to the job but, realizing the medics were in trouble, went balls out for them. A paramedic could ask for no greater tribute.

As the patient was moved, he screamed in Polish, "Pain," clutched his chest, then went into V-Tach, a deadly rhythm. He was unconscious, no pulse. His wife fainted, his son screamed, and one partner ripped the patient's shirt open and applied the two gel pads. The firemen stood aside, stunned. Once the patient was hooked up, one medic screamed "Clear" as the EMTs pushed through the crowd. The medic charged up the Physio Control Lifepak 12, ready to discharge two hundred joules of electrical current through the man's chest. In a split second, he delivered a bolt of energy more powerful than the energy in the electric chair. The medics hoped not to jump-start the heart, but to stun it for a nanosecond. That would be enough to let the heart's natural pacemakers reset themselves. His partner yelled, "Clear!" Although it was a cold winter day, both were soaked in sweat. One yelled "Clear" two more times and hit the discharge button.

Suddenly there was an explosion! Smoke followed a blinding electrical arc. The smell of burning flesh permeated the back of the bus, as the patient's arms lunged grotesquely upward. It appeared to the family that their loved one was in agony, reaching for his chest. They screamed and the firemen ducked. The paramedic's heart was in his mouth as he asked if everyone was okay. One EMT was with them. Although in shock, his partner brought the other back to the job at hand.

"I have no pulse. What's his rhythm?" he asked.

"The same," he said, reaching for a second set of cables with trembling hands. The salt of sweat burned his eyes. As his partner started ventilating the patient, he ripped off the destroyed cables, cursing and setting up a second set. The EMS command directed all paramedic units to carry two cables for such reasons. In the split second it took to set up everything, both cursed the system for the piece of shit they were working with.

The EMT, without having to be asked, removed the destroyed pad with pieces of burned flesh on it. With the cable and pad replaced, the medic called, "Clear."

The EMT left the patient's chest and the medic released the Bag Valve Mask. It was hooked up to the intubation tube he had placed with precision, as he sat, squeezed between the patient's head and the captain's chair. He was breathing for the lifeless patient.

"Clear," yelled the medic at the chest.

Two more times he yelled, then, hit the discharge button. This time it worked. He converted the patient into a sinus tach—fast heart rate. The paramedic's right hand, the EMT, said the patient had a pulse and was trying to get a blood pressure. His partner drew medication to protect and keep the patient in this rhythm. The EMT told them the pressure and asked for the keys to drive the bus. His partner was herding the distraught family to the second bus. The son wanted to ride in this bus to "make sure you don't kill my father." The paramedic reached over to close the door. One fireman, wearing an EMT patch, finally reacted by helping close the door and herding the distraught family member to the other bus. The medic told the EMT to wait until he could see the other EMT get safely into the front of their bus. Once in, the EMT acknowledged the paramedic's silent concern by waving.

"Okay. Let's go!" his partner yelled. As the buses pulled away, the firemen were standing in the street, shaking their heads. While working on the patient, the medic heard the EMT call for a notification so the emergency room staff would be ready.

The EMT was told, "Stand by, unit. I'm trying to give out a sick job." The dispatcher lectured the EMT, "Notifications are a courtesy. Furthermore, you were not assigned the job. I have you out with no radio response. Now what is your notification?" he asked sarcastically.

The information was transmitted and a patrol boss decided he would go to the hospital to "talk with that unit."

At the hospital, the staff complained about not receiving a notification.

"Well, I'm notifying you now," said one paramedic.

Later, both ran interference with the boss who wanted to do a charge package because he did not like the EMT crew. After cleaning up and restocking, the crew went back to the base for new monitor and cables, along with paperwork. The lieutenant behind the desk only wanted to be left alone. He tried to discourage them from doing the write-up.

The following week they were called into QA (Quality Assurance). They were not told why, just to report. The pressure increased.

The doctor said, "You are not in trouble but . . ." It seemed this doctor spotted the ACR. He wanted to know why the crew did not call and ask for Valium to intubate the patient. They told him the whole story, orders, explosion, and all. He agreed the other doctor made some strange requests, but he did not want to get into it. The doctor became silent, dead silent.

A certain female paramedic student was called out of class and provided transportation to a hearing. It seemed that one day a while back, her partner, who had many years on the job, noticed she was really stressed out. She, being new, had seen a lot in her first month, and he knew she was not handling it well. He figured she needed some cheering up, so he drove her to Central Park. That's in Manhattan; they were a Queens unit! There he led her out of the bus, rented a rowboat, and took her for a relaxing ride. The sunlight danced across the lake, turning it into a magical sea of sparkling, bubbling, pearls. As she lay back in the boat, the healing energy of the sun cut through her tense body. Like gentle yet strong fingers, the energy worked its way through her clothes, into her body, to her soul. Her spirit was rejuvenated. She heard the birds sing. The air was filled with nature's scents, perfume from the flowers and nearby trees.

Her partner saw the change as her body melted and he started to paddle back. She got back into the bus with a soft tender smile and drove away.

Unfortunately for the crew, there was a police department internal affairs unit in a building across the street. They had set up a sting to nail police officers, but became interested in the parked EMS unit. At first they figured the crew had a job in the park.

When the crew got in the rowboat, the heroes of internal affairs kept the tape rolling. They sent the tape to EMS. The girl was responding to an act of kindness, not forgotten, that had happened long ago. Once in front of the judge, she realized the levity of their discretion.

Her partner, realizing her aspirations, convinced the judge to let her off easy. He was the old-timer and as such took responsibility, as well as a hefty hit. She became a paramedic.

An academy paramedic instructor noticed an ad in the local paper concerning White Castle's fiftieth anniversary. White Castle made these small, mouth-watering hamburgers that were unbelievably delicious. The paramedic decided he would treat his staff friends to a feast.

At the local White Castle, he ordered a gigantic box filled with hamburgers. Behind him was a local TV news crew filming the anniversary. Seeing a paramedic buying that many burgers, they realized they had their story. As the paramedic turned to walk out, both arms supporting the gigantic box overflowing with burgers, he was stopped. The reporter explained her dilemma and requested the paramedic's assistance. New York paramedics and EMTs were always willing to help.

After the camera was in place, the lights adjusted, the reporter started her interview. As the paramedic lifted the heavy box off the counter, the girl behind the counter beamed. Standing sideways while talking, his white, orange and blue paramedic patch filled the lens as the cameraman homed in on it. The interview went something like this.

"Gee, I see you like White Castle hamburgers," said the reporter.

"Yes, I certainly do," he responded, lifting the box off the counter, paramedic patch centered.

"As a paramedic, how do you feel about eating the meat and its associated damage to the heart?" the reporter asked.

Always able to think on his feet, he replied with an impish smile, "Well as you can see, all this grease goes through the arteries and lubricates them." With the interview over, he returned to the academy to share his feast.

Later that night the phone rang off the hook. Dr. Dario Gonzalez, Medical Director for Clinical Affairs, had completed a tough day. He turned on the TV and to say he was emotional would be an understatement.

We had never known Dr. Gonzalez as one who either cared for us or was professional. New doctors going through EMS rotations had confirmed this more than once. They had repeatedly told us of Dr. Gonzalez's demeaning statements about paramedics.

The disgruntled doctor's game was to rule by fear and intimidation. During the medic oral exams, he'd grill the student, sometimes up to two hours, cursing and crushing the new medic. This happened to Julio Marrero as well as others. The student failed and was re-examined in front of a different doctor and passed. The doctor's peers knew and disliked what he was doing, but none would stop him. With each new class, he fed his overinflated ego.

We dealt with such stupidity by improvising. A seasoned crew would always outwit a dispatcher or doctor. In the old days, we checked out our archaic telemetry equipment by transmitting an EKG to ensure the system worked. One crew got fed up with this nonsense. One medic hooked up his partner and transmitted the strip. The doctor at the other end was heard to say, "Holy shit." Then asked, "How is this showing at your end?"

"Fine," responded the medic. "What's up, doc?"

"Are you sure it's fine?"

"Yeah. I have a perfect rate of seventy-six, and perfect normal sinus rhythm. Why?"

"Uh, nothing. Guess it's this damn equipment again. Out."

It seemed that the doctor was receiving an EKG with a rate of about thirty-eight, extremely slow since the average is between eighty and one hundred. The doctor thought it was the machines. In reality it was the paramedic's resting pulse. He was a long distance runner and his heart was finely tuned to provide the optimal pumping with the minimal of strain. Telemetry didn't ask for more strips and our two heroes went for coffee. So much for all that book learning against the common sense and tenacity of a street-smart NYC paramedic.

Serving a richly multifarious society, I've experienced weird (to my crew members anyway) cases involving supernatural forces. Some extremely healing, others banefully destructive.

The supernatural was nothing new to me, but it amazed me how people used their metaphysical talents to hurt and destroy, instead of adding to creation.

Having been taught by fantastic healers, I became both a Reiki and Karuna Master. As a teacher and practitioner with international credentialing in biofield medicine in this country, I've had some interesting experiences with my partners like Tom Reynolds which could fill another book. Instead I'll just state that I've used my gift with paramedic Charlie Liccese who witnessed total surgical pain relief on a sixteen year old girl. Paramedic Brian Keegan saw the results on a brain damaged blind South American infant, and another medic witnessed the results with a full blown AIDS infected crack using prostitute who was a critical asthmatic. She had been intubated seven times leaving the hospital on Friday after the latest attack. We picked her up that Sunday night. All our Western medicine failed to work and she refused to be intubated by shaking her head though unable to talk, leaning forward like a tripod, getting tired —basically, 'circling the drain,' or dying, for you gentle readers. Bouncing in the back of the unit, setting up the tube kit and hearing that little voice singing that song Knock, Knock, Knocking on Heavens Door I asked if she wanted me to "try something?" When we pulled into Lincoln Hospital the doctor asked why we called a notification since she was speaking and breathing perfectly.

Paramedics Anthony Gorman and Dan Huie witnessed an SVT (Supraventricular Tachycardia), which is a heart rate above 150 beats per minute, broken. The patient's rate was 176 beats per minute and failed to respond to Adenosine administered via IV and wasn't unstable yet to use electricity (Synchronized) Cardioversion. There was no underlying A-Fib present showing on the 12 lead EKG. While paramedic Gorman called for Diltiazem to be used diagnostically, I did my thing since a good twelve minutes had passed and the life of Adenosine is 4-6 seconds. Suddenly the woman said; "You're doing it to me." Then I heard a "Holy shit!" from Dan who was watching the monitor. Her heart rate went from 176 to 86, then remained at 84. So I was nicknamed

'Voodoo Jim' by Anthony, which was also my call sign when I first went to Bosnia. In an earlier case, he along with a home aide witnessed relief to a 95-year-old with pain caused by fluid leakage of incorrectly placed IV in a hospital before they sent home to suffer. The Aide jumped back after she felt the energy become ice cold, just what was needed for swelling.

This story will also demonstrate that there are no isolated cases, or chance meetings. Indeed when a butterfly flaps its wings in Japan the breeze is felt here.

"Fourteen Boy ten-ninety-eight (available)," the EMT said into the radio.

The crew rolled out of their garage at Metropolitan Hospital at Ninety-sixth Street and Second Avenue in Spanish Harlem. It was a crisp, autumn Sunday morning. The sun's bright rays inundated the buildings with a vibrant, clean energy. Adorned in a colorful pageant of leaves, the trees stretched toward the powder blue sky.

Greeted by Rolando Chavez, the crew picked up their coffee and hot bread from his landmark La Alegria bakery on 103rd Street. Later, finding a spot near the East River, they read the Sunday papers, as a tugboat lazily pushed an oversized barge up the glittering river. One of the crew looked up. The river had a peaceful, majestic energy to it. The sunlight sparkled on the crystal blue water like little beads of pearls. The wake of the passing boats created white foam like a Sapporo beer poured into a cold glass. To his right, he noted a man peacefully fishing. Smiling, he returned to reading.

His name was Wakeem. He was a feared drug dealer in Harlem. Thirty years old, his six-foot, thin frame was crowned with a narrow face. Unkempt dreadlocks flowed past his shoulders. A mid-range drug dealer on the rise, he had a following of users, prostitutes, and white adventurers. He was renowned for spiritual possession and intervention in the mixed Caribbean-African community.

Several weeks prior, he had been at the Green Light Club, where he was insulted by one of the owners, Angelo. His bodyguard Angel wanted to kill the "White Devil" right there on the dance floor. But Wakeem saw a different road to take. He accepted the insults and waited. Time was limited to this plane of existence. The spirits were eternal. He ordered his Angels to get information concerning the "White Devil." Revenge would be slow, painful, and deadly.

He laughed as he thought, *The White Devil will pay in ways he will never suspect, until it is too late.*

Wanda rolled over in her bed, finding her sister, Ada, cuddled next to her. The fourteen-year-old twin must have had another bad night, since she crawled in with Wanda.

Bad nights developed into bad days for her sister. Ada had been released into her mother's care from school on Friday after becoming emotionally hysterical in class. The doctors at the local clinic and the school psychologist agreed it was because of the messy divorce between the girls' parents, Yolanda and Angelo.

Yolanda confided to Wanda that Ada would grow out of the tantrums. But it wasn't happening, Wanda thought, as she looked at her sleeping sister. Ada had always been the more sensitive one and had unseen friends. During the last few months, she appeared to be going mad, seeing strange things.

Their mother took Ada to see numerous doctors at King's County Hospital and other hospitals in the area. All the doctors thought the disease was a delusional disorder and wanted Ada in a hospital, on a drug regimen. The mother refused. She preferred the diagnosis of the clinic and school.

As the girl's condition worsened, the mother requested help from a "Spiritual Cleanser." He owned a botanica in Brooklyn. Yolanda did not believe in the spirit world, but she would do anything to keep her child from being institutionalized. She gave him a chance.

The date was set and the "Cleanser" arrived. The mother had a violent argument with Ada the day before and grew more frightened by what she saw and trusted people less and less.

Yolanda stated flatly, "The 'Cleanser' will arrive and work on you, with your full cooperation." Moving her hand to caress her daughter's jaw, she continued, "Unless, Ada, you want me to listen to the Western doctors, dooming you."

Ada agreed.

Arriving at the neatly kept apartment, the "Cleanser" asked for and accepted the family's donation before he started. Next he cleared the apartment of "all evil spirits."

Looking at Yolanda, he asked, "Are there or were there any people in your life who would wish harm to you or your daughter?"

"No," Yolanda answered uneasily.

"While cleaning the apartment did any of you find anything or pick up anything found in the streets?"

"No," she answered with a chuckle. At this point, she wondered if she had made the correct decision in asking for his help.

"Do you or your daughters dabble in voodoo, witchcraft or obeha, black magic?"

"No." This question sent a shiver up her spine for some unknown reason.

The "Cleanser," a Dominican, performed a ceremony that involved bathing Ada, lighting candles, and the use of an egg, coconut, and cornmeal. Another concoction of herbs was placed on coals and the incense billowed, surrounding Ada's naked body.

Hours passed. Finally, he applied coca butter to the girl's hands, feet, chest, and back as she lay on a cloth-covered kitchen table in the living room. When he finished, he had her stand.

She stood before him, her mother, with sister behind. Ada's shoulders hunched forward. Gaunt and naked, her ribs stuck through anemic skin. The girl's head bowed. A tear formed as her mother looked at the tortuous, stooped mass of flesh that was once her vibrant daughter.

The "Cleanser" reached over, raised her head, and looked into Ada's eyes. For the first time in weeks, a gentle smile crossed Ada's face.

Suddenly, he felt a chill of death in the air. The windows were closed, yet everyone felt a sudden, cold breeze enter the room. Yolanda frantically looked around the room, as Wanda grabbed her. Their hair and clothing rustled in the ungodly chilling breeze. Fear gripped the "Cleanser" as he grabbed his chest, profusely sweating. His shirt and pants were drenched with perspiration.

Yolanda stood in shock as she watched his clothing become soaked and his skin turn snow white. Suddenly, the breeze was gone, but where? Where did it come from? She reached for Wanda, who was frozen by the sight. All now felt the chill.

Ada continued to smile.

"I must stop. I must stop! This spirit is too great," the Cleanser screamed in horror.

Since Ada's back was to her mother and sister, they never saw the smile. As the Cleanser backed away from Ada, she lowered her head, the smile gone. The Cleanser ran from the apartment.

He was last seen alive entering his botanica. His body was found the following day, an apparent suicide. That's what the police said, finding the donation sticking out of his mouth.

The unit responded to "Three Three Charlie you have an EDP" (Extremely Disturbed Patient, or Everyday Person as the crews say). At the apartment, one of the EMTs tripped on the doormat. As he went to replace it, he saw a strange graphic glyph. Thinking it was a cute good luck symbol, he centered the mat on it and entered the apartment.

Inside, the crew found the mother with the police officers. She wanted her daughter, Ada, committed to Brookdale Hospital.

When the EMT interviewed the mother, she confided in him about her doubts and use of "The Cleanser." Yolanda explained that though she was raised in a traditional Dominican family, she did not believe in spirits, good or bad.

Wanda helped put a coat on her frail, frightened fourteen-year-old twin. The crew talked to Ada, but she mumbled, "I see a skeleton in a river swimming, attached to a wire."

"Who is it?" the EMT asked.

She looked at the EMTs with fearful eyes. Attempting to talk, she said, "I think . . ." but never completed the sentence, lowering her head.

The EMT raised her head, looking into her eyes. He saw the difference and knew she was possessed.

The girl and her family were transported without incident to Brookdale Hospital.

It had been a fast-moving, wild night at The Green Light. Money, drugs, deafening music, and flesh rolled. Wakeem sat drinking his beer. Angelo, the White Devil, approached him. The angels stood by.

"Hey, I thought I told you last month I never wanted to see you here again, asshole." Wakeem slowly looked up from his drink. His blue, piercing eyes made contact with Angelo's.

Angelo, looking like a mad Danny Devito, couldn't look into Wakeem's eyes. He felt an electric shock jolt his body. "Ha, but I be here on a mission to ask you a question, man."

"Yeah," said Angelo, getting a weird feeling and pulling his sharkskin pants up on his potbelly waist.

"Yes, man. I wanted to ask, how is Ada?"

Angelo was shocked as Wakeem stood up from the table, looking no longer into his eyes, but through him to his soul.

"Get the fuck out of here, now!" Angelo screamed. He tried to throw a punch, but was grabbed by his own bouncers.

Wakeem leisurely finished his drink, looked at Angelo, smiled, and walked out. Angelo scratched himself, as his skin felt like it was crawling. He stormed across the floor, shoving patrons on the way to his office. He wiped the sweat from his face and picked up the phone.

"What the fuck you mean she's in the Brookdale Hospital?" Angelo screamed into the phone.

"Listen to me, bitch, if I find you have not been taking care of her, I'll kick your . . ." The phone went dead.

The next morning, Angelo went to see his daughter. He was a short, plump man. He wore a cheap gray suit. Around his neck was an initialed silver cross and chain his mother had given him. He hid it, but did not get rid of it because he believed it was a good luck charm. His expensive gold watch and diamond ring flashed his importance.

As the elevator climbed to the floor, he knew something strange had drawn him here. He shrugged uncomfortably, as his skin started to crawl. Empty handed, he entered the waiting room, flashing an angry glance at Wanda and Yolanda. He was escorted inside to see his daughter.

She sat alone at a table in the sterile visiting room. Her long, unkempt hair hung down her shoulders. She sat looking at her hands. Ada wore a blue-and-white hospital gown open in the back but tied at the neck. Slippers covered her small feet. He approached the table and sat. The room, no, his daughter, had a disgusting, unclean smell to her.

"Ada, Ada," he said. He nervously looked around the room. Slowly he reached with his hand. Applying pressure to her jaw, he raised Ada's face and looked into her eyes. He was searching for an answer, not for Ada, but for himself. He always resented the twins and hated Yolanda for having them. They cramped his lifestyle.

Her brown eyes were lifeless and sunken into two dark holes. Her lips were dry and cracked with blood. Her skin was as white as her gown and peeling like a bad case of psoriasis. She hunched forward, looking ninety instead of fourteen. As he observed her, a mysterious chill went through him.

"I'll kill that bastard," he muttered.

Suddenly, Ada's eyes came alive. She smiled. Her teeth were coated with a yellowish film. A strange, deep Jamaican accent and putrid smell came from her mouth as she said, "I will make you a dead man."

Angelo jumped up from the table, almost falling backward, sending the chair flying. "You're fuckin' sick!" he screamed, grabbing his head.

Security ran toward him, as he looked at his daughter who bowed her head and played with her fingers. Ada's smile was gone forever.

As security started to escort him out, Ada turned to him.

"Papa," she said in a normal, but shaken voice.

Her father bent closer to listen.

"It's you I see swimming in the river."

She returned to playing with her cracked fingernails. Angelo was physically assisted as he screamed, "What river? I can't swim! You psycho bitch!"

Once outside, he gained his composure and looked at Yolanda and Wanda.

"I don't know what you two have done to her, but when I find out I'll kill you both."

"Sir, let's go." The two large security guards assisted him into the elevator and stood beside him until he walked out the front door.

"Guess it runs in the family," one security officer said to the other.

Saturday night had been good at the club. No one had seen Angelo, but they understood his daughter was in the hospital. He probably needed a few days off and would check in Monday.

As for Wakeem, his apartment had four people ready for a "service." He stood in his room, adorned in a long-sleeved, black silk robe, awaiting his disciples to be made ready. Each wore an article of clothing the color of his favorite saint. Tyrone knocked on Wakeem's door and silently escorted him to his place of honor. All knelt face down until he sat. Seated on the oversized pillow in the candlelit apartment, he looked around.

The soft light caressed each face. To his right sat Tyrone, one of his angels. In front of him sat Tishshawn, a twenty-year-old ho. Next to her sat her friend, Veronica, a twenty-two-year-old mother of three. To his left sat Leticia, a nineteen-year-old girl from Honduras. She had been drawn to his services by her wish to gain power from the spirits.

The room was small, but clean. African artifacts hung from the walls. A small, multicolored rug in the shape of the African continent adorned one wall. A radiant painting called *Shaman*, done by Guillo Perez as a tribute to the natives of the Caribbean, hung on another. The rich kaleidoscope of colors exploded, giving the apartment a dignified gaiety. The partition dividing the living room from the kitchen had several large green plants.

Everyone sat on large floor pillows in silence. Attention was on Wakeem, as he raised his right hand. His expensive gold watch glittered in the candlelight. His large diamond ring magnified the soft light, sending laserlike streaks across the room. He snapped his fingers and Tyrone got up and bowed to him.

Tyrone brought out the small altar to the god Yoruba (thunder god) and placed it in the corner of the living room. Next, after bowing to the altar and Wakeem, he went to the kitchen. There he lit several candles on the platter and placed the hooded object in the center. He walked into the center of the room and placed the platter on a rotating wooden platform that sat about six inches off the floor.

Once Wakeem gave the signal, the cover was removed and the platter rotated slowly for all to see. The centerpiece was the head of a black female. The light from the candles gave her jet-black, oiled hair radiance. Her lips were large and her red lipstick looked glossy against her dark skin. Dark eyelashes accentuated her brown eyes. Even in death, with her eyes sewn open, she looked fearful. A blood-spattered butterfly clip adorned her hair. The face stared hauntingly at each person as it turned ever so slowly on the wooden platform.

As the service continued, they passed around the cocaine crack pipe. Its smoke drifted endlessly as the head continued to rotate.

"Fourteen Boy. Report of a Jumper Down," came the call, breaking the quiet of the tranquil Sunday morning. The crew packed up their papers, the coffee and hot bread long since devoured. They turned on the emergency lights and hit the siren as they pulled onto a near-empty First Avenue heading North to Harlem. Several minutes later, they pulled onto the block of brownstones. A sector pulled up behind them. Both crews got out and stretched, not seeing anything.

Suddenly, from across the street in a hallway, a woman stuck her head out the door and screamed, "Over here. We need help here."

The police and EMTs started toward the hallway. The iron fence in front of the location was splattered with blood and clothing. The second floor window was open, with the curtain ripped and hanging out. One EMT went with the two officers, guns drawn, and entered the building. The other EMT headed toward the screaming woman. Upon entering the lobby, he was met by three women trying to comfort a fourth.

"He is going to get me. Oh my God. He is going to kill me."

The EMT yelled, "Everyone, shut the fuck up."

All except the one screaming became quiet. "What's going on?" he asked.

"After hearing the shots, I saw her jump from the window," one woman stated. He looked at the patient.

"Are you hurt?" She kept babbling about the guy trying to kill her, then started to scream. It was too early in the morning for this. The EMT gave her a quick slap across her face, bringing her to her senses.

"Where are you hurt?" he demanded to know.

The jeans she had been wearing were ripped, and as she spread her legs, blood flowed.

"Strip. Strip now," he said, realizing it was she who landed on the iron fence. If the steel penetrated her femoral artery, she would bleed to death in a few minutes. If the bleeding was coming from her vagina, he didn't want to think about it.

The girl, with the assistance of the woman, stripped naked from the waist down.

"Spread," he ordered. He found what he was after. The iron fence did indeed impale her through the femur, the upper, thicker part of the leg. He was amazed to see an entry, and exit point, still bleeding. Realizing she was as high as a kite, he stood up and looked at her.

"Hands above your head. Now, keep them there."

He ran his hands under her sweatshirt across her chest to her neck then down to her naked waist. At the same time, he ran his other hand up her back to her neck and back down. Not finding any blood, he was satisfied there were no other gaping wounds. As he applied a trauma dressing, another unit arrived. He turned the patient over to them and proceeded across the street to find his partner.

He entered the brownstone, and as he approached the door to the apartment, he noticed a strange graphic glyph above it. Upon entering, he turned left past the half kitchen into the living room.

"Holy shit. Holy fuckin' shit," he heard the officer say. The EMT stepped around the officer. There was a black male dressed in a black silk robe, holding a pistol in his right hand, a crack pipe in his left, dead. To his right was another male, dead. In front, by the open window, was a girl, dead. To the left, slumped on the floor, was a younger girl, dead. All were shot between the eyes. In the center of the room rotated a human head, its mouth contorted into a smile. The room was deadly quiet. A nauseating stench of evil and death hung in the air.

The EMT walked with the cops to the other unit and the girl. She was paranoid and pleaded for protection from "him."

They learned that after the service, the drugs as well as the sex flowed all night. At sunrise, when the magic pipe got to the leader one last time, he produced a nine-millimeter and shot everyone in the head. Most were so stoned they didn't realize, until it was too late. The patient, Tishshawn, realized what was happening and bolted out the window, grabbing a curtain to slow her fall. The curtain broke and she became impaled on the fence, six feet above the ground. She got free and headed toward the first person who came to her aid.

"One Oh Zebra. Stress Free, you have an 'unconscious.' The crew wondered what this unconscious would prove to be. Most in this city were anything but unconscious. NYC EMS was so good at triaging calls. Right. We know it can be anything from a dog bite to a drunk, to an unfounded. The job wasn't an unconscious until we made it so. According to the text, the people on the scene refused to do CPR. The crew realized the patient was dead. Just how dead remained to be seen.

The bus pulled off the FDR Drive heading north near the Madison Street Bridge, which crosses the Harlem River. It traveled through the low brush, heading down toward the water. The crew saw the lights of the fire truck and a Basic bus with EMTs from Harlem. The crew parked and got out.

It was a beautiful autumn evening. A harbor unit pulled up to the dock. Two elderly black gentlemen stood by, talking to the cops, one with fishing pole in hand. Finally, the body was reeled in. It was a skeleton. Its hands were tied behind its back with rope. An initialed silver cross and chain were stuck in the bones around the neck. The two elderly men had been fishing when one of them hooked the unconscious. He only pulled it in so far, before he realized what he'd caught and dropped his pole.

Wanda had been having bad dreams as had her mother. Ada was still in the hospital, doing even worse. As Wanda cleaned the apartment, she never noticed the dark, stenciled, graphic glyph drawn into the tile floor under their beds.

The Chinese community was an honorable and closed culture. We had to work hard to win the trust of these people. It was on this basis that the following story was recreated. The names have been changed, but the incident was as real today, as when it happened years ago early in my career.

Chan sat in the park across from his house. A meandering, crystal-clear stream babbled peacefully past. Before him were the majestic Rocky Mountains. Here no one knew him or his children. Life was good. A car pulled up and he saw his eldest child get out. She was so beautiful. Walking over without a word, placing her arm around him, she saw the first ever tears slowly run down his cheeks. Chan kissed her softly, wrapping his arm around her. They both realized their insignificance in comparison to the beauty and vibrant energy of Mother Earth. He held her pregnant body close.

How had he gotten to this point? How far had he run across this world? he pondered.

It all started so long ago.

The United States in 1945 would drop an atomic bomb on Hiroshima. In a spilt second man's blinding insanity evaporated, or burned to death, over 70,000 women, children and men. Several days later, another bomb would incinerate Nagasaki. Yet, America would conveniently "forget," and would give carte blanche freedom to the butchers of Japan who wantonly slaughtered, tortured, raped, poisoned, and depravedly killed over 500,000 women, children, babies, men and elderly in one action, in one city: Nanking, China. The United States sold its honor and memory for the results of "secret" experiments on Chinese civilians and Allied and American POWs. With the stroke of a pen, the State Department and Presidency of America blotted out any trust, and honor won by its servicemen in World War II for "medical" concerns gained from the darkest depths of perversion. The ramifications of this disgraceful betrayal are still very palpable in the Chinese psyche today, both here and there.

It was 1937; a bloodthirsty crimson war cloud descended, then swallowed Nanking as the carnivorous Imperial Japanese Army devoured its occupants. A small village sat several miles north of the city. Food was scarce, but not fear and total disbelief as delirious, emaciated skeletons of humanity escaping the city blindly wandered the roads, babbling of inconceivable atrocities. Japan's infamous Unit 731 was conducting genocide via "doctors" against the Chinese civilians. These doctors were evil incarnate, conducting autopsies on conscious patients!

Chan was ten and lucky to live away from the main city out in the country. The family had a small plot of land they tended. One warm morning, Chan, frightfully startled, bolted from sleep to the harsh cracking sounds of gunfire and his mother's screams. Running to the window, he climbed out, hiding in the bushes. Several soldiers and an officer of the Imperial Japanese Army were in front. They were screaming that a Japanese patrol had been ambushed by the Chinese Army and they were tracking down the culprits. They demanded information. A crazed soldier held his younger brother, Xan, four years old, by his hair. Frantically screaming, his mother implored for mercy.

Though small and gaunt in stature, the Japanese officer's large, glazed eyes menacingly peered behind thin black-framed spectacles. Intoxicated from the bloodfest in Nanking, he nervously wiped the excessive perspiration on his soiled uniform sleeve. A furious, vengeful expression contorted his thin face as the woman begged for her son's life, repeating at a fever pitch that the whole family "respect authority!" With one hand on his large saber, he signaled two helmeted soldiers, who then stripped and took turns raping her in the dust as she continued to plead for the child. When the deed was done, she knelt before them naked and bruised. The morning sun was hot, the surrounding jungle steaming, the dusty ground dry, fine and powdery.

Suddenly lurching toward the officer, shrieking, "We respect authority. Please—" She was caught midway with a rifle butt knocking her to the ground. Xan screamed, attempting to kick the officer. On command, the mother was pulled by her hair to a kneeling position, to observe her young son's throat slashed from ear to ear. The victim struggled, twisting in the air, his small hands unable to stop the tidal wave of gushing bright red blood. His body shuddered before going limp. As the soldier released the child's hair, Xan hit the dusty ground with a deadly thud. Finally, the wailing mother was shot. Her naked body collapsed into the dust. One of the soldiers kicked Xan like a soccer ball, onto her. Both blood-splattered, sweaty yellow bodies lay in death's grip. As the dust settled, both the temperature from the blazing sun and the soldier's fiendish laughter rose.

Approaching the house momentarily, Chan slipped undetected into the jungle. He looked back only once, observing the bodies in the dust, their blood now silently mixing on the ground. White smoke bellowed lazily from the shack as red and orange flames lapped at what was once home. Moving deeper into the lush jungle, he only heard the crackling of the blazing dried bamboo.

Avoiding both the Japanese and Chinese patrols, he hurried into the small town to find his father, older brother, and cousin. As he approached, he realized something was very wrong. Shots were mixed in with horrific screams. The smell of fires reached his nose once again as sweat burned his stark, horror-filled eyes.

In the town, he cautiously moved to the factory to find his father and brother.

Japanese soldiers were everywhere. With their bayonet-tipped rifles glistening in the sunlight, they harshly rounded up everyone, herding confused, petrified girls and women into the center of town. Children were torn from their mothers' arms and slaughtered by gunfire or bayonet. The men were hustled toward the open field near the Yangtze River.

Chan hoped his father and brother had managed to hide in the factory. Upon entering, he froze. Twenty men and boys were stripped naked, hanging upside down with their hands tied behind their backs. They hung silently from the factory conveyor hooks. All had been shot or bayoneted to death. Their life-blood splattered the concrete floor where it mixed with the oil and grease, turning dark. He did not see his father, brother, or cousin.

He continued to search, moving through the jungle, working his way in the shadows toward the river. Chan was almost captured, as a crazed Japanese soldier chased two girls into the jungle. The soldier furiously bayoneted one from behind. She abruptly stopped, stood erect, struggling as petite, slender fingers savagely tore her blouse open. A terrifying expression of confusion contorted her young lotus face. An agonizing whimper succumbed to a primordial death rattle escaping parted lips as she saw the silver tip protrude out four inches between two naked breasts. The tip disappeared in a bright, violent, volcanic eruption of red blood as she fell forward, collapsing onto the lush green jungle floor, landing two feet from Chan. He stared, not releasing a tear. Lifeless eyes filled with agony hauntingly stared at him. Motionless hands held her chest, where the bayonet had exited. It appeared to Chan she was holding her heart. The only sound from the girl was the bubbling of blood coming from the subsiding flow of blood between her breasts.

Slithering away from the dead girl, he proceeded to skirt the tree line, remaining in the shadows. Finally, he was in position. The Yangtze River was a backdrop to the clearing in front of him. Wiping his eyes of sweat, he saw a group of five men and boys being led to the bank of the river. His older brother was among them. With arms tied behind them, they were made to kneel. Several Japanese soldiers and officers took photographs, cheering as each victim was bayoneted to death. It was a game to see who could kill his prey the fastest. Chan's brother fought with his legs, rolling on the ground, parrying several bayonet lunges. His screams penetrated Chan's covered ears as the bayonet entered his right leg. The crowd applauded as the soldier now thrust the bayonet deep into his brother's stomach. Chan watched, no longer covering his ears as his brother, still moaning, was kicked off the bank into the body-swollen river.

Suddenly, he heard his father's voice. His father shrieked frantically at the officer, demanding an end to the insanity. "We respect authority! We trusted your word to live in peace, protected by you. We respect authority."

The officer raised his hand and the crowd became still. He took Chan's father to the center of the clearing, near where Chan was hiding. His father was made to kneel. Chan saw dead bodies up and down the bank of the river; others moaned from mortal wounds while being eaten by large, savage, hungry rats.

His father, accepting his sentence, knelt with the sun hot on his back. The Japanese officer drew his sword. "I will now show you respect for Japanese Imperial Army authority," he whispered. As the sword cut through the boiling, humid air, the officer screamed, "Banzai!"

In a millisecond, the head left the body, rolling to a stop about eight feet in front of his son. The officer kicked over the body that now spasmed lifelessly on the ground as his troops joined in a thunderous, frenzied roar of "Banzai"! The bloodfest continued.

As the head came to a halt, Chan's father's eyes were still open and saw his son hiding directly in front of him. He attempted to yell to him, but his mouth would not move. His vision was becoming blurry as he saw a rat come close. It knocked his head to the side as it started gnawing and eating his right eyeball. He screamed a silent scream. His vision was getting blurrier as he saw the boy crawling away. Chan would grow up never shedding another tear. The last thing his father saw was another rat pouncing on his face.

Years later, in a distant land, American scientists would learn that the brain remains alive for six to eight minutes before the cells start to die from the lack of oxygen.

After the war, Chan bought his way to America, paying an exorbitant amount of money to Chinese smugglers. He worked long hours in sweatshop conditions to pay off the twenty thousand dollars with interest. Yet, he managed to put money away, realizing one day he would need it.

His cousin, who had survived the massacre by the Japanese, found him in New York's Chinatown. Both worked hard and lived with two other families in a three-room apartment near Mott Street. These were hard but good times.

One day, his cousin returned home beat up and slashed. The older woman had called 911, much to the fear and indignation of Chan and his cousin. Two officers entered first, followed by two men dressed in different uniforms. The officers were losing patience and had passed several derogatory statements when the cousin would not cooperate in giving them information.

Chan noticed that the other two uniformed people showed actual concern for his cousin. After spending several days in the hospital, his cousin spoke to the detectives who followed up on the case. Chan listened as they promised "protection" if the cousin would give them the names they needed. After all, mused his cousin, *This is America. Here, authority will protect me.* Chan was not sold on the idea. He asked his cousin many questions about the other uniforms that had worked on him. All the cousin could say was they were like doctors, showing concern, honorable people.

A week later, Chan returned to the apartment to be told his cousin was dead. The police described it as a suicide. The official report was that he was homesick for China so he threw himself off the roof of the building.

Chan knew better. He would write his cousin's family telling them of his death.

Over the years, as the family of his late cousin continued to write, his fortune became better. He was free of his debt, owned his own business, and was about to bring Mia, his bride, to America. He had sent a dowry for her and also paying men to smuggle her to America. She proved to be a devoted wife.

After several more years, she gave him two daughters and a son. His business boomed and he moved his family to a beautiful home in Queens.

Across the street was a wonderful park with a man-made lake. His children brought him and his wife honors. Good fortune smiled upon them as his business grew. He opened a new shop and received honors from the Chinese and Korean communities of Flushing. Life was good. His oldest daughter, Teresa, graduated Pratt Institute in the fall as an accountant. His twelve-year-old boy, Xan, was interested in sports and science, a straight A student. Tai, the youngest, at age nine, showed much promise in gymnastics, receiving many awards and trophies.

But all was not well.

Recently new leadership had taken over the leading "transport company" that smuggled people from China to America. The members of this gang of Fuzhonese were younger, violent, and not honorable. Their reputation preceded them. Their leader, Zen, had found Chan's wife's name in the inventory list and made the connection when he saw her fare had been paid outright in American dollars.

With two of his associates, he had visited Chan's home. They were respectfully met until Chan realized it was a shakedown. They wanted part of his business, claiming it would pay for the interest owed for bringing Mia to America. Chan would have no part of it, ordering them out.

As they left, Chan stood by the front door. The peaceful, tree-lined park turned ugly as the smell from a neighbor's barbecue hit his nostrils. He smelled the smoke and realized his world was burning again.

Zen, on more than one occasion, approached Teresa at the university, or on the street in Flushing. She put up a brave front, but was repulsed and fearful of the little greasy man. Months had gone by. Mia had wanted Chan to go to the authorities, but he forbade it. He did not even trust banks, hiding large sums of money in the house, in case he had to run again. Months went by and things were going well. Perhaps, thought Teresa, Zen had gotten the message, as she pushed the creepy fear of him out of her mind.

It was a beautiful autumn day when Teresa approached the front door. She wore a navy blue skirt, white silk blouse, blue jacket and black high heels. Her silk black hair was in a ponytail, adorned with a jade hairclip. A black band watch adorned a slender wrist, with a jade bracelet. From her neck hung a small jade loop on a dark gold chain. She sang to herself walking to the door, retrieving the mail. It had been a great day, with a successful interview at IBM and TRW. Both firms wanted to hire her once she passed the coming accountant exam. Entering the house, she didn't hear her mother's desperate warning through duct tape. When she did, it was too late.

"What?"

"Well, come on in, Teresa," Zen said.

One of his associates shut the door behind, giving her a gentle but firm shove toward Zen. Looking into the gaily decorated living room, she saw her mother tied to a high back chair. Duct tape covered her mouth.

"What are you doing? Get out!" screamed Teresa, attempting to run to her mother. This effort was rewarded by a stinging smack across the face, as one of the associates grabbed her. The mail went flying, as did the jade loop on the gold chain. It lodged itself in the corner by the door. Teresa was hustled into the living room, close to her mother.

The rug was a soft royal blue. Sun shone through the large bay window. A crushed velvet couch with colorful pillows filled the room, as did family pictures, and fresh flowers in a hand-painted vase. The girl was held by the larger associate, as Zen, much shorter, approached her. He wore a suit, shirt, and tie, all black. His black hair was as greasy as the stubble on his chin. He wore black sunglasses.

Her breathing increased as she saw his frightful sneer.

"Want to go out with me now?" he asked, smiling.

"Go to hell," Teresa bravely retorted, as her mother screamed through her gag.

Zen slowly ran his hand up her chest as she squirmed. The silk felt good under his hand, but her firm breast felt even better. Being shorter, he stepped forward to kiss her. She twisted her head, unable to release herself from the grip of the associate. Zen grabbed her hair, pulling her head to the side. Holding it with one hand, he viciously tore the delicate blouse open with the other. Her eyes suddenly bulged in fear. Forcefully, he kissed her lips. In a desperate act of bravado, she spat in his face. He signaled for the other associate who had been standing near Mia. He grabbed her long, black hair, eliciting a yelp as her head shot backward. With her in this position, Zen finished ripping the blouse and stood on his toes, starting to kiss her chest.

With back painfully arched and head thrust back Teresa struck, crashing her knee into his groin. He screamed in agony, doubling up on the soft lush rug. When he regained his composure, he slowly stood. "Still defiant?" he queried. Her head rose to look at him, her eyes glaring, but also reflecting a trace of fear he immediately spotted. *Indeed a sensual sight,* he thought to himself.

"I will enjoy you later. We will have an electrifying time. You will be my model for your family. You, my love, will pay." He suddenly snarled, and his rock-like fist smashed into her soft stomach. The total fury of the impact surprised the men holding her as both released her as she hit the floor in agony.

"Tie her!" he commanded.

Continuing to feebly struggle, she was rolled onto her stomach, removing the blue business jacket. Teresa was easily subdued. Her hands were tied behind her back, then her feet, stripped of her shoes after attempting one final kick. Finally, duct tape covered her mouth. She saw her mother in the chair crying, as Zen massaged her now exposed breasts.

"Since you do not want to go out with me, Teresa, I will take you for a little walk anyway," he said in a foreboding laugh.

She struggled as he looped a length of rope between her tied feet and started to drag her toward the cellar stairwell. Across the living room floor, she continued to twist, trying to free herself and see her mother. Onward she was slowly dragged into the kitchen where she saw him open the door. After turning on the light, Zen looked. He enjoyed the total commanding power he was experiencing even more than the view. Teresa didn't matter, it could be any one of his many victims. What mattered was the thrill from the power. He proceeded down the stairs, giggling, dragging his prize behind him. Slowly, step by step, he dragged her down, each step eliciting a moan. When he was at the bottom, he forcefully yanked the rope, sending Teresa crashing off the last four steps onto the concrete floor, knocking her unconscious.

When she awoke, she heard voices, but was confused. She could not see nor speak. Her hair seemed to be hanging above her. As she remained still, her consciousness became more lucid, the voices clearer.

"I want you to release my family!" she heard her father demand.

Then she heard a crack. Now it was all coming back to her. Her ankles and head hurt. Zen had knocked her unconscious, dragging her down the cellar stairs. Now she was bound upside down by her ankles from the pull-up bar her father had set up for Xan and Tia. He had turned a large portion of the basement into a gym for both. She twisted to free herself.

"Ha, I see your daughter is awake now," Zen said, as he ripped off the blindfold.

In silence, she observed her father, badly beaten, bleeding in a chair. Next to him sat a very frightened Tia. Her brother Xan was standing tied to a steel support beam. He wore only his dungarees. He also had been beaten. When her eyes were able to focus, she saw her mother gagged, breasts exposed, tied in the same tall, back chair, looking at her. Teresa's legs and head ached. The silk blouse was torn open, hanging down and covering part of her face. Her favorite navy blue skirt was now hiding nothing as it hung down, exposing lavender bikini panties. With both feet tied far apart, legs spread wide, she felt vulnerable.

"As I have told you, old man, you owe me money. Now I have gone out of my way to show you, even with this calculator, how much you owe me," he said, holding a pocket calculator in his hand.

"I am a businessman. As such, I expect respect and payment."

"You are a thief on the same scale as the Japanese," Chan yelled, before receiving another blow.

Mia screamed through the tape.

"Get the tape off her," Zen ordered. "Now woman, what do you want to say?"

"Please! Please we respect authority! If we owe you money, then please I will work for you. Please remember your mother. She taught you—"

Before she could finish, Zen lunged at her, smashing her swollen face.

"My mother! My mother!" He insanely screeched, grabbing her hair and thrashing her head from side to side. "She was weak. I am not! Now where is the money?" he screamed, terror filling the old lady's eyes. Releasing her, he slowly walked over to Teresa, shaking to regain his composure.

He knew well the mentality of the Chinese family and its pride in their eldest child. He would exploit this to get to Chan. He also had a deep hatred for this girl, who would not feed his ego. But using Teresa to get to Chan was only part of his plan. He relished in the glow of both physical and mental degradation. Zen would receive more fulfilment from cherishing Teresa's agonizing and begging to stop hurting than sex with her. He had no idea, however, that the harder he pushed Chan, the deeper he would recede into a dark past. Nor could he know the deep devotion and inner strength of Teresa. Slowly, he ran his hand between Teresa's legs.

"Where's the money?" he screamed. No one answered.

"Okay," he took out scissors. Everyone recoiled in horror thinking he was going to gut his prey.

"Let's see what your daughter is hiding."

As Teresa twisted, he proceeded to cut off pieces of her clothing, stopping after removing a piece to admire his work, posing for a quick snapshot. When he was finished, she was hanging, naked. Smiling, he pulled out a knife. Teresa's almond eyes were filled with terror. She attempted to squirm away, screaming into the duct tape. Zen grabbed a handful of hair and put the knife to her slender throat. The doorbell rang. The mother screamed, but the three men laughed as Zen went upstairs. He let in two more members of his crew. Downstairs, they set up the video equipment and opened some beers.

"Last chance, old man. Where is the money?" Chan did not move.

Teresa saw her brother and sister looking at her. They just stared.

"We'll do the girl first," Zen said.

Teresa's muscles tightened when they grabbed her baby sister.

"No," she screamed through her gag, violently shaking her head.

"What? Want to play now?" Zen asked.

Teresa, broken in humiliation, slowly nodded her head, tears falling to the floor.

"Isn't that wonderful?" he said, slowly walking next to her. "Now she wants to play."

They all chuckled.

The camera was going as the second one was being set up. He stood beside his captured, naked, inverted, hanging game running his right hand up her velvety back. It glided to her buttock that he felt go taut.

"I'll loosen that up later," he giggled. A thick sense of doom became palpable and permeated Teresa as huge terror-filled eyes pleaded. Next, his fingers played with her exposed vaginal area. Teresa squirmed.

"Give me one of those," he said, and an associate handed him a cold beer. "How's this look?" he asked, resting against her. His left hand holding a beer, while his right hand was behind her right leg, violating her vagina with his finger for all to see.

"Great," they all said, laughing.

Soon all could hear the moist, slurping sound as his fingers played between her legs. Chan, like the rest of his family, was mesmerized. Not only were they captured physically, but mentally. Xan, Tia, and Mia watched as Zen drank his beer posing for pictures as he inserted his finger, then fingers, finally bottle, into Teresa's vagina.

Chan saw it happening again. He was a young boy inside the plant, where the bodies hung. Teresa stopped twisting, hanging in shock and humiliation. She looked at her family. All eyes were on her as an uncontrolled quiver chilled her body. The once gaily painted and decorated gym basement now took on a cheerless, morbid aura. All except her father were crying. He sat stoically, lost in a surreal meditative trance. It was as if he was looking right at her, yet through her.

Is this not bothering him? What is wrong with him? What is he doing? Teresa thought for a moment, suddenly finding herself outside her body, observing herself!

I must be going into shock, she heard her mind say. But, just as confusing, she heard a voice, her other voice, softly say, *No, you are not.* Teresa shook her head, trying to clear it.

"Ha, look," Zen joyfully exclaimed, moving the bottle. "She's really getting into it."

He and his associates laughed, not realizing what was happening. Teresa shook her head again, to bring herself back to reality.

But then the voice asked, *Which reality?*

Then she heard Zen's voice. "Well, Teresa, you'll have to wait. You had your chance for enjoyment for now. Now it is time to share."

He removed the bottle, stepping away from her, licking it. Realizing what was to come, she twisted and screamed into the tape. Tia moved obediently, eyes filled with confusion and fear as they brought her to the ping-pong table.

Hours passed as the cameras filmed. Sexual abuse was perpetrated upon each member of the family. Then humiliation followed as each terrified family member was forced to perform acts on each other. Through it all, her father remained stoic, even when performing acts. This was not missed by Teresa, who wondered if this had anything to do with the war. She knew he had a deep hatred for the Japanese. By nature he was a man of few words. The only time she was released from the bar was so she could be "serviced" by her family members. The only time the tape was removed from her mouth was to service them. Teresa, terrified, followed her father's lead, stoically performing the acts as ordered. The only emotion shown was tenderly helping her petrified siblings perform on her.

Finally, it was all about to come to an end, but first the promise. Teresa was now repositioned, hanging from the bar in a sitting position. Her doe-like eyes frantically shot from man to man then Zen as electrical wires were attached to her breasts. Her body glistened from sweat. She wailed uncontrollably as cold beer was poured slowly over her to get a better reaction.

"This will be an electrifying experience for you, Teresa."

Demonic laughter turning into a hideous howl filled the basement.

Terrified, she let a mournful, muffled whimper escape her covered mouth as Zen inserted and secured a contact into her vagina. A paralyzing panic swept Teresa as the shadow of death became a reality as the final contact was inserted in her anus. Teresa was lost, all hope crushed when the first shock struck. The body jolted and convulsed under the voltage. Even after the switch stopped sending electricity cascading through her body, the fiery spasm of unworldly agony continued. Now panicking in dreaded anticipation, Teresa screamed into the tape begging, pleading for mercy, agreeing to do *anything*. Zen smiled. "I promised you an electrifying time and I keep my word," he chuckled as he held the switch up for her to see. He looked deeply into her cowering eyes. He laughed as her body tensed, then shuddered as he pretended to hit the switch. Her head fell forward, body still trembling. Reaching over, he pulled her haggard head up. "Okay, I won't disappoint you," he cheerfully said. Another excruciating wave bolted through her with the force of a hundred typhoons. Teresa looked ninety years old, hanging from the ropes. Her jet-black hair was soaked from the sweat. All bladder control was lost as she urinated on her brother who lay unconscious under her. Zen, a true sexual sadist, consumed the fragrance of desolation, relishing the total wanton destruction observed in Teresa's despondent eyes.

Suddenly, she looked upon herself once again from the outside.

Her other self stood naked, radiant, with a flower in her hair. *You are learning a powerful lesson,* she whispered. Teresa raised her head to see herself.

"You really did it this time," one of Zen's associates remarked, laughing.

All silently watched as she appeared to be totally in a world of her own.

There was a soft, unspeakable beauty to her other self's body. The altered self slowly brought both delicate hands reverently together in prayer, looking serene. Silently, Teresa prayed, not knowing if there was a God, but needing one. The voltage savagely tore into her body, causing it to uncontrollably trash as the muscles alternated between tonic and clonic movements, the agony draining the last of glimmers of life. *Surrender, the key to survival. Surrender, become one and live.* Her body quaked and thrashed as Zen laughingly increased the voltage.

Many years before, her father had been in the park with her and had explained, "See the baby, how soft he is?" He pointed to a new baby lying on a blanket.

"Look at the old man," pointing to himself making her giggle.

"See how wrinkled I am?" She nodded.

"Now look at this dead piece of wood. Is it hard or soft, child?"

"It is hard, Father," she answered, looking serious.

"As you grow older, you will be involved in many things, situations, problems. Sometimes even love will cause pain. The key is to remember to be like the new tree in the storm and bend. Become one with the storm, the energy, and you will survive. Fight it, and you will wind up like this dead, hard piece of wood."

"Pain is no good," the child remarked, remembering both her humiliation and punishment she received for lying once.

"Pain *is good*," he whispered, drawing her close, "it reminds us to be obedient. Obedience in turn is the foundation of life." With this, he tickled her. The child's laughter filled the lush park.

"But, Father, are you obedient?"

"Yes, indeed. I was very obedient to my parents," his voice drifting off. "And we must all be obedient to nature," he said, cupping a flower, both smelling its soft fragrance. "This is the *only* way to harmony and to learn the lessons pain brings us."

As her body bolted back and forth, she heard herself command, "Become one. Do not fight the energy. Do not fight the pain. Become submissive, obedient, one with it. In harmony you will find true freedom, and learn its lesson."

Thrashing in her ropes, Teresa attempted to do exactly that. She stopped thrashing, fighting the anticipation. Suddenly the agonizing pain was a discomfort. What was she learning?

What is happening?

Another jolt hit. She could hear Zen and the others laughing as her back grotesquely arched in hyperextension with extreme muscle rigidity, yet that was only a physical appearance.

Now a man stood before her, dressed in a white robe.

"Suffering is caused by opposition, a belief in separation and the refusal to receive. It is increased by efforts to escape. Accept, my child. Become obedient, be one."

Her attention was drawn to his chest where his heart appeared! Red flames erupted from it. "These are flames of searing love for you, Teresa," he softly said as her physical body continued to react to increased voltage. "Open your heart and live."

Then Buddha appeared within the flaming heart, growing, consuming "the man" who disappeared within the golden Buddha that now sat before her, smiling. Without a word, the Buddha now disappeared between the breasts of the smiling, radiant girl who stood before her. Teresa now *knew* the Christ-Buddha were one, as she and this girl were one. She also *knew* all were within her heart.

Suddenly, she saw a man on a cross. As her body wretched and thrashed uncontrollably, in the ropes she surrendered while straining to concentrate on what was appearing. All at once, it exploded into a bright, dazzling supernova of warm light. Her heart filled with a joy, as she had never known. As the light dissipated, the joy didn't, as she started to feel the pain in her body again. *This time would be different,* she told herself. Just as she became determined to totally surrender, the next jolt did not come. Wearily, she raised her head, looking at her father. Their eyes met, Chan knew.

"I will give you the money," the unbroken man said, realizing he needed to get out of the basement if his family was to be saved.

They helped him stand, pulling up his blood-splattered shorts and pants. As he was escorted to the stairs, he looked back to see his family.

Mia was unconscious, slumped in the chair. Tia, naked, was still tied over the pommel horse. Xan lay unconscious under Teresa. He had performed as ordered, but received a final, brutal beating for trying to protect her from the electrical torture. His arms were tied behind him, lying on his side. Even the warm urine he now lay in had not brought him out of his unconsciousness. His naked, young body reminded Chan of his brother lost long ago.

For a split second, he looked at Teresa; their eyes met again. A slight smile appeared on his face. Then he turned. Teresa was silent, looking down at her brother. She did not know if she would ever see her father again or if the family would survive. But she knew what he had taught about acceptance. Thus, whatever was to happen, she would accept. And for the first time since this nightmare started, she knew she was free from the ego's fear.

Chan took Zen out to the garage where he had one of two safes built into the floor. Once Zen had the money and his "associates" were all accounted for, he smashed the old man goodbye. Hours later, Chan awakened and hobbled down the stairs.

For a week, very little talk took place inside the house. Each time the phone or doorbell rang, the family jumped. Mia had enough going against her husband and family's wishes contacting the authorities.

A report was completed and stuffed away. There was no evidence and no one would corroborate her story. A black detective, after receiving no help from the family, walked out the door, when something caught his eye. He bent down and retrieved the small jade loop and gold chain.

"Yours?" he asked, as he looked at the young girl.

"Thank you," Teresa whispered, looking down.

As he walked to the car, he knew in his heart something had happened. But without help, without trust, he could do nothing.

The sad part, he thought to himself, *I understand the fear and lack of trust. I only wish they understood how badly I want to help.*

After the detective was gone, Mia, for the first time in her marriage, screamed at her husband and family, "This is America! We respect the laws. We respect authority. They will protect us if we step forward."

Her plea fell on deaf ears in her family, but others were listening.

I was on overtime when we responded to a call of "Person Shot."

As we pulled up, there was a woman lying next to the family car. She had been shot in the back of the head. We covered the body with a sheet. I made eye contact with the elderly Chinese gentleman. In a split second we looked, *and* understood. We had both seen this before, and we both recognized each other after all this time. Now the elderly man stood stoically as he was asked questions by the police officer, while Chinese neighbors stood by the gentleman.

Finally, in frustration, the officer said, "Don't you people know we are trying to help you? Talk to me," he demanded.

The old man looked at him, saw me shake my head, fully understanding.

"We respect authority," he uttered softly.

That was the last he said or allowed his family to say. Several weeks later, as I drove past the house on the quiet, tree-lined Queens street, it was empty.

It was several years later before the New York Police Department would attempt to build inroads into the Chinese community. Unfortunately, much work remained. The society, as a whole, remained closed to non-Chinese. That was a shame since they had so much to teach us.

In all the years working Stress Free, I knew two things. If we got a call in Chinatown, it was legit. The folks never called unless it was beyond their ability. Secondly, once on the scene, we had to make the connection with them. Realizing we respected them, their medicine, culture, and doctors, they proved to be the most gracious people I have ever met.

As a society we have come a long way, but not far enough. As EMS, we have pushed the envelope of cultural barriers in dealing with patients. This was the only job where people would hand off their wives, mothers, daughters, or sons for us to work on. Yes, society would always have that one percent who remained ignorant. But they could be taken in stride when we realized the trust my brothers and sisters had built. I spoke for all my brothers and sisters in NYC EMS as well as others in America, and all over the world when I said 99.99 percent were people who care. They were honorable people indeed.

SIX

Special Ops, Special Moments, Special People

One unique aspect of being an EMS paramedic in midtown Manhattan was that New York City was the epicenter of the world. It was the greatest social experiment in the history of mankind, the melting pot of America. As paramedics, we met the world's rich, famous, and bizarre.

We would find ourselves in a DPU (Dignity Protection Unit), riding in a convoy with the president or vice president of the United States, or riding coverage with a dictator, tyrant, or prime minister. It was fun to be listed for this interesting detail.

I was once part of this detail for President Bush, as well as other dignitaries from around the world. As with everything else, the quality control was no longer there, as you will read concerning the president of a Balkan nation and the wannabe EMS chief whom we all love, yeah.

But first, let's stop and see how Paramedic Bubba and Paramedic Schrang handled a crisis in the Waldorf Astoria.

Paramedic James Patrick "Bubba" Fallar and I were out of the bus and in the office at Bellevue, about to turn in the narcotics, when the call came in. The dispatcher told us to say nothing on the radio, just to read the text.

In the unit, we brought up the job on the screen. It stated we were to go to the Waldorf Astoria where the Secret Service would meet us. We would then be escorted to the wife of the president of an island country in Europe, who was having difficulty breathing.

As we pulled onto First Avenue heading north, we wiped the sleep from our eyes. The traffic started to build on this crisp, clear Friday morning. We saw an EMS captain and lieutenant in the command car ahead of us. They too were assigned the sensitive job.

Once we pulled a pair (10-88), we were met by our American Secret Service. These guys were cool. They were as underpaid as we were, yet their professionalism and humor were second to none. They also had a better style and approach to situations than the FBI (Famous But Inept). The latter couldn't find a hooker in a house of ill repute with a hundred-dollar bill.

We were ushered into the secure elevator. Neither of us said a word until we got to the suite. Entering, we were halted by the patient's own security. As we waited, the door opened and in walked the captain and a lieutenant. The captain stood about four feet in width and shorter than five feet in height. She and I had a long, rocky history together.

She was arguing with security about their right to be there.

I said, "They're with us," and turned back to talking with the Secret Service agent.

While we were talking, a man with a doctor's bag walked by toward the patient's room, saying, "Hi guys."

"Who's that?" I asked the head of foreign security.

"Oh, he's a doctor," was the reply. At that point I'd had enough.

"So your first lady is having difficulty breathing and he walks by with a bag? Why are we being held here?"

"Oh, but sir, he's a doctor," he replied.

I blurted, "Well sir, the fact is, we, NYC paramedics, are better than doctors. As you can see, our bags are bigger." Hit them with the visual. People believe what they see.

"That's correct," replied the Secret Service agents.

"When our president is in town, these are the guys who ride with him."

"Thanks, guys," I said.

"I'll be back in a moment," said the security agent and then disappeared down a long corridor to the bedroom.

Upon the gentleman's return he said, "Please follow me."

As we started down the corridor, the Captain "Munchkin" and the Lieutenant "Prozac" were stopped. I turned to see Bubba chuckling, as both of them looked for help once again.

"They are here to assist us," I said, turning away, starting to laugh since I could sense their frustration. They were on the scene to act as our resource and control the scene. But the only scene created was by them. They had no jurisdiction over patient care unless they saw us killing the patient. Since both officers were EMTs, they wouldn't have a clue if we were killing the patient. Technically, they were our bosses. So why not work with them? Besides, it was always good to have extra hands to carry the bags.

I followed the security officer in the lead. As we approached the bedroom, I heard the doctor say to the patient, "Don't worry. These EMS people just want you to sign a paper. Once that's done, they will get into their ambulance and leave."

As we entered the gigantic bedroom, I saw an older gentleman seated on a high-back chair against the wall by a window. Security agents stood around the room. The morning rays bathed the room in a glow of serenity.

The patient was an attractive woman in her fifties. She was sitting up in an enormous bed, resting against oversized pillows. She wore a lacy, lavender nightgown on which was offset her white hair. She was covered to the waist with a colorful blanket of spring flowers and birds.

As I entered, pulling our stretcher loaded with equipment, I looked directly at the doctor and announced, "The EMS people are here." He stood up and approached me.

"The president's wife has not been feeling well today. She had some shortness of breath before you came, but now she is fine. She's willing to sign your paper so you can leave."

"Wrong," I said, hearing Bubba moan. He knew what was coming and it would surely be a humiliation to this unsuspecting doctor.

"What do you mean wrong? I said we do not need an ambulance."

"What are her vital signs, doc?"

"Uh, they're fine."

"What are they?" He looked at me with anger in his eyes. I continued, "Perhaps you can answer this one. Did the patient have chest pain and does the patient have any history of medical problems?" The doctor's discomfort showed and the patient smiled.

"Uh, no, I don't believe chest pain and no medical history," he said in a huff.

I looked at Bubba, who was smiling and said, "Lets see, no vital signs, a questionable chest pain story, no prior history. Thank you, doctor. Please stand over there." I pointed to a spot by security. One of their agents reached out and helped the doctor to the spot.

The patient had a radiant smile on her face.

"Hi there," I said, kneeling on the bed, reaching with one hand to touch hers and the other to rest on her shoulder.

"Hello," she responded, her hazel eyes sparking in the light.

"I'm Jim and the short guy there is Bubba. We are NYC paramedics, not ambulance drivers, and we would like to check you out. Is that okay with you?"

"Oh that would be wonderful," she replied. Bubba was already in motion getting the blood pressure cuff out of the oxygen bag.

"Bubba is going to take your vital signs, blood pressure, pulse, and listen to your lungs while you and I talk. Okay?" She nodded, looking at Bubba climb up on the bed to get access to her arm.

"Are you having any problems at this moment? Difficulty in breathing, chest pain, or dizziness, anything?"

"Oh, no, I'm fine now."

"Okay. Why don't you tell me what happened?"

She stated something woke her out of her sleep. She couldn't breathe and although there was no chest pain, there was discomfort, like something was wrong. It only lasted for a few minutes and then she caught her breath.

"Did you do anything that helped?"

"Oh yes. I prayed."

"That's always the first and best thing to do," I said with a smile, as she squeezed my hand. "Did you move around? Did this feeling in your chest move around?"

"Oh, I sat up and then started to feel better."

"I bet you propped a number of pillows behind you, huh?"

"Oh yes. They are beautiful, aren't they?"

"Ah, typical woman noticing the pillows," I said as she laughed. "Did the discomfort move any?"

"No."

"Okay, with one finger show me where it was." She pointed at her sternum in the center of her chest. "What did it feel like?"

"Like something running over my chest." I reached over and applied some pressure to her chest.

"Does this hurt?"

"No." I saw Bubba about to listen to her lungs. He had already given me her vital signs which were good, although her pressure was slightly elevated.

"I want you to take a deep breath for me, while Bubba listens to your lungs, and tell me if it hurts?"

She complied, without any problem. She explained she never had anything like this happen to her and she wanted to get on with a shopping spree before leaving for Europe the next day.

Bubba looked at me. "Jim, got some very fine rales at the bases. Take a listen, please."

I listened, and sure enough there were some rales, indicating fluid in her lungs. Something happened to the heart, which acts like a pump. When working correctly, it pumps the blood throughout the body. With an electrical or musculature problem, the latter, usually the left ventricle, the fluid backed into her lungs, awaking her. When she sat up, gravity from Mother Earth pulled down, assisting her by creating a fluid shift. That's why a lot of elderly patients will say, "Jesus saved me. I couldn't breathe so I got up, knelt down and prayed to Jesus. In a little while I could breathe again."

"How are you feeling now, young lady?"

"Oh, I feel fine now that I'm sitting up."

"That's great to hear. Right now we are going to do an EKG—that's a look at your heart, okay?"

"Sure."

When we completed evaluating the patient, Bubba and I realized she had to be seen in a hospital. We saw atria fibrillation—A-Fib on the monitor. I looked at the strip, the Lifepak 5. This, unlike the current Lifepak 12, could not do a 12 lead, but it was certainly more reliable than the 12. Think of it in these terms: The 12 lead looks at the heart completely, as opposed to the 5 lead—in parts.

The doctor wanted to get into the act.

"Let me see that," he demanded. I just stood there, looking at him, and he got the message, "Please."

"It's only A-Fib," he sarcastically announced to the room, trying to put us down.

"That's correct, doctor. Undocumented A-Fib. No former history, A-Fib. Thus I want her seen at a hospital to have a 12 lead done at the minimum."

"She can have that done in my office."

"And where is your office?" I played along with him.

"Downstairs."

"Wrong," I said. Bubba was enjoying this as he sat with the patient on the bed.

"What do you mean wrong? I'm the doctor."

"We are the paramedics. Since she has a new rhythm, if you would like, you can bring your machine here. The patient will not be exerting her heart going anywhere."

He looked at me and says, "But the machine is heavy."

"Then you can take one of the staff members from the hotel to help you." He started heading toward the door when I said,

"Oh, by the way, doctor."

"Yes?" I too have a 12 lead at home. It's made in Japan and very compact. Perhaps you should consider buying one."

He spun around, almost walking into the door buck as he left. I could hear our two supervisors grabbing their chests.

We turned our attention back to the patient and explained to her that we were going to give her an aspirin and start an IV in case we had to give her any medication. She agreed. So here she is, in bed with two burly paramedics.

"I don't want you going back to your country telling everyone you were in bed with two New York City paramedics." With that she got hysterical.

The Prozac Queen was taking a hit and the captain was holding her up to keep her from hitting the floor. Bubba got the IV. We had her packaged, IV, oxygen, and monitor, when the doctor walks in.

"What are you doing?"

"We started patient care and will be taking her to a hospital for further evaluation," I said. The older gentleman, seated in the chair, spoke before the doctor could say a word.

"Excuse me, sir." We all looked at him. "Sir, what is your recommendation?" he asked.

"Excuse me, sir, but may I ask your relation to the patient?"

"Certainly, I'm her husband. The President."

"Nice to meet you, Mr. President. My recommendation is that she be further evaluated at a hospital. She wants to do some shopping before you two fly back to your country. You will never hear the end of it if she is shopping and strokes out. You know how women are."

He smiled, understanding, "She will go to the hospital. Now which one would you recommend?"

"Bellevue, NYU, New York, they're all good. But I want her seen."

"Our president has a suite in Bellevue, Mr. President," said a Secret Service agent.

Now the doctor had to get into the act. "I want Lenox Hill." It seems that this is where he worked when he wasn't moonlighting at the Waldorf Astoria.

The president looked at me, "Would that be fine?"

"Okay." Off we went. The threat potential for the president and his wife was low, otherwise, we would have opted for Bellevue. On the way, we had the highway cops on their little bikes along with the Secret Service and the president's security force riding with us.

I have always had this mental block concerning "The Hill" (Lenox Hill Hospital). It's located on Seventy-seventh Street between Lexington and Park Avenues. Aside from it definitely not being one of my favorite hospitals, I always think it is on Seventieth Street. So this morning I was about to break away from the convoy, when my little voice said not to.

Boy, am I glad. I could see the headlines: "NYC Paramedics Kidnap President's Wife and Agents."

We pulled into Lenox Hill and brought in the patient. Inside we were shoved aside, not by the Secret Service or the president's security, but by the Lenox Hill staff. We were cut short on our presentation as the good doctor chimed in. Standing off on the side, I waited for Bubba to stop smiling at the nurses and finish the ACR. The head of the president's security approached me.

"Sir," he said, pulling out his checkbook and pen. "The president and I wish to thank you. We do not have such a service as yours in our country. How much do I make the check out for?"

I looked at the Secret Service agent behind him who was rolling his eyes. I was trying hard not to laugh. Instead, I looked the agent in the eyes, smiled.

"Sir," I said to the president's security, "that will not be necessary, since I know the hospital will bill you. It has truly been our pleasure to serve you."

"Thank you so much," he said.

I was walking out when the agent caught up to me. "Nice going."

"The care or turning down the gift?" We both laughed. When Bubba heard about it, he almost died. He had visions of a holiday in the islands with the girls, his wife and daughters, of course . . .

The following is based on an actual incident that took place at the United Nations. Identities have been changed to avoid an international incident and to protect *Ricky,* who told me this story, but all personalities, or lack of, will be recognized by those who worked Battalion 8 at a specific time in history.

Sometimes things didn't fall into place. Indeed, for one aspiring captain, a wannabe chief, this was the case. The situation deteriorated fast upon meeting Mr. Murphy of Murphy's Law Firm.

In conducting operations, one struggles to succeed against both known operational problems and the element of the unknown. We the crews were good tacticians, using KISS (Keep It Simple Stupid) for our planning and adding to the equation Murphy's Law. The law states: "Whatever can go wrong, will go wrong." The same can't be said for EMS managers.

In New York we pulled special details for dignitaries as well as at various sensitive locations, such as the United Nations. As leaders of the world gathered, a certain captain, from *Bellevue,* was assigned the UN for a week. It was a beautiful autumn day; the air was crisp as his chauffeur, an EMT named Ricky, drove him up to the security booth on First Avenue. The United Nations police officer waved him in.

Getting out of his command vehicle, he stretched his stringbean body and took a deep breath, suddenly choking from the diesel exhaust as his aide pulled away. He took a puff from his asthma pump. Embarrassed, he quickly wiped his sweaty face and put the pump away as his aide returned. His chest, now fully able to expand, filled with pride, as he realized there were no EMS chiefs in the area. He was the one who stood between death and destruction if something happened. Yes, things had changed since he was nicknamed "Lollipop" in the South Bronx by the *girls* he visited while on patrol.

He had a background in SOD (Special Operations Division). Having run numerous operations in the past, he felt confident in handling anything. His chauffeur/aide could only imagine the thoughts of false grandeur running through the young captain's delusional mind. Having an aide by his side only added to his feeling of self-importance.

As he turned to enter the building, his aide carried the officer's cheap black canvas bag with several radios protruding out and held the door. Before entering, the captain turned, observing the paramedic unit in place with two medics. He smiled, turned, and glided through the door, followed by his aide.

Walking through hallowed halls of the "Glass Building," he relished his job. This day he would be rubbing elbows with people of power. Such an assignment would aid in his quest to be chief. His ultimate goal, of course, was to be Chief of EMS Command.

The oversized female medic decided to help herself to lunch in the cafeteria, leaving her dorky, sloppily dressed partner in the unit. He had recently been upgraded to paramedic from EMT. Since the fire gods gutted the EMS Academy, EMTs and paramedics could no longer claim to be the finest EMTs and paramedics in the world.

She, on the other hand, had been at various facilities. She could not intubate or start an IV, which presented a problem, especially for the patient. But the Fire God was concerned only with quantity, not quality.

The mentality was easy to understand, considering education was not a priority for the firemen. How much education is needed to order someone to put the "wet stuff" on the "red stuff?" Oversimplification, true, but understand that neurons dysfunction in a synaptic gap polluted with smoke and testosterone even with education. But EMS was worse. The chiefs who ran it had GEDs—no management degrees—and were EMTs.

In normal people, the synaptic gap is clear until a chemical messenger is released, going from one side of the neuron to the other, rendering a reaction. In the Fire God's head, without a guideline from one side of the synaptic gap to the other, the signal would never get there. If the responding messenger is not wearing a Scott Pack filled with oxygen, no one knows what the messenger may produce, if it even gets to the other side. Thus when dealing with firemen, and fire gods in particular, you need to demonstrate both professional knowledge as a paramedic and a deep sense of compassion for these handicapped souls. Concerning EMS chiefs and wannabees, you just shake your head.

Back in the unit, both medics had volunteered for the HAZMAT (Hazardous Material Unit), thinking they could pick up easy overtime. Both were snatched into the unit, because any medic who had been around awhile wanted nothing to do with Fidney's "Mop and Glow" team. The once-prestigious knowledgeable units were reduced to wearing their yellow "condoms" (Level A Protective Suits) when Fire felt they should, or taking blood pressures and pulses of firemen, if the firemen wanted.

The medic gathered her feast and wandered back to the unit. Luckily, her partner didn't take up too much space, so she could spread out her goodies on the dash computer/radio console and still hold a tray of food on her lap. As she opened her Diet Coke, she smiled at the smell of the freshly cooked pork.

Her partner continued to sleep. His worn-out Playgirl baseball hat was pulled down over his eyes. He looked so cute, she thought, with his long, gold earring dangling to his shoulder. Only a glimpse of his brightly dyed orange hair could be seen. A red bandanna around his neck and tucked into the front of his uniform shirt hid the tattooed swastika on his throat. He told her it was a symbol of good luck through the centuries, having had it placed on his throat, believing it would prevent him from saying foul things and bless all he ate.

Reaching for the plastic fork to scoop up gravy-covered mashed potatoes, she looked at the tattoo on his right hand and realized that the gravy wasn't the only thing hot. As the food disappeared into her mouth, she felt he was meant for her.

The captain stood in the corner of the room with his numerous radios on. One of the security officers walked over and asked him to kindly turn them off. In the command section, no one needed to hear what the fire department or Manhattan EMS units were doing. The other radios blared out their SOD jargon. The radios were turned off, as several other Secret Service types frowned at the captain.

Outside, several Secret Service men ran to the bus. "We need you upstairs," they said to the medic as she sipped her Diet Coke and knitted. "The president is having difficulty breathing. It may be a heart attack!"

"Sorry," she said, placing the Diet Coke down on the dash, "we are HAZMAT." As they stormed off, she continued, "We don't treat common patients. We are . . ." They were gone so she went back to her knitting. The agents ran toward the entrance, yelling into their sleeves.

She looked over at her partner and decided to make him a new scarf.

Downstairs, there was a flurry as the captain waited for his aide to bring him a cold drink. The young EMT was cornered outside the room and asked, "What the hell is a Hazbeen?" He thought it was a joke and started laughing until he saw how deadly serious they were.

"Perhaps you gentlemen should talk to my captain," he suggested and started walking into the crowded room. The captain's focus was on the large, frosty *Orange Crush* drink. Being observant, he never noticed the human wave of Secret Service agents surge behind the EMT.

"Sir—" Before the EMT could complete his statement, the captain went into a tirade about why it had taken so long to get his drink.

The Secret Service agents had enough, blurting out, "What the hell is a Hazbeen unit? Or Hazbat?" they demanded.

The young EMT, being street smart, stepped aside and moved away from the captain. He observed him, now relishing his drink as well as the attention.

"Let me explain, gentlemen," he pompously started, "in the beginning, EMS didn't have such . . ."

Before he could finish, one large and impatient agent screamed, "Look, asshole. Is it a fuckin' ambulance or not?"

"Why yes, of course it is," the confused captain answered.

"Then why the fuck were we told Hazbats don't touch patients?"

"What?" yelled the captain, spilling his drink on his white shirt.

"The president is upstairs having a fuckin' heart attack and we need an ambulance now!"

"I'll get one! What floor?" Given the information, he grabbed his driver and headed out the door.

"Walk slowly," he told his aide as he picked up speed. Once outside, he turned around and raced back into the room again. At his table he picked up his radios, took a fast swig of the Orange Crush, and headed out the door. Running across the hall, he tried to contact Manhattan Central but was told to "stand by." Once again, he was told, "Standby, I have a sick job to give out." It never dawned on the captain that this was the crap the crews had to go through each day.

Finally, he said, "This is Captain So and So. I need an ALS unit to my location forthwith!"

Meanwhile, our wannabe chief and "hope I'm still a captain at the end of the day" stood in front of the HAZMAT unit, shrieking at the top of his lungs. After literally jumping up and down, he noted to his dismay that neither medic was looking at him. He banged on the window. Slowly the female rolled it down. He continued to scream, but she didn't seem to mind. Then, she turned off her CD player and took out her earplugs.

"Did you say something, sir?" she asked.

For the third time, he went into his tirade, instead of dispatching the crew to the president. The female started to blubber.

"You're not a nice man. We're going in as overtime personnel!"

It finally dawned on the captain that if they went in as overtime personnel, he would not have anyone for the . . . *Oh my God*. It hit him, "The president!" Profusely sweating, the Orange Crush spot becoming larger, he frantically apologized, now begging the medic to get her partner, equipment and follow him. After she dried her eyes and checked eyeliner, she woke her partner, and they followed the fast-moving captain. The captain's aide saw where this was going and walked several paces behind the captain.

The captain introduced himself to the patient, who was from Europe. The Secret Service pulled him aside.

"Let the medics check out the president," one burly agent uttered.

As the female medic stepped forward with the blood pressure cuff, her partner approached with the ACR. The captain, never a man to miss anything, spotted the unauthorized baseball hat.

"Get that off," the captain said with gritting teeth.

"But sir, didn't Chief McCracken go after you for an unauthorized 'Gator' hat? Didn't you continue to wear it?" asked the medic.

"I'm giving you a direct order," the captain said, as he reached for the unauthorized blue hat with naked female on it. The captain pulled it off, developing rapid shortness of breath. With the hat in hand, he clutched his chest, staring at the medic's bright orange hair and gold earrings. The captain leaned against the wall as Ricky figured he would shortly be working an arrest—his captain's. Quickly, he reached into the captain's pocket for his Albuterol pump.

"Deep breaths, sir," he said, holding the pump to the pale, diaphoretic captain's blowfish-type lips. "Good, sir. Continue to suck on it." Ricky's Spanish accent was pronounced and everyone in the room, including the president, looked at him.

Unperturbed, the female medic read off the vital signs, sensuously smiling at her partner. The president was getting worse. Not from his heart condition, but from what he was witnessing.

"Sir, your social security number, please?" the medic asked. The Secret Service looked at each other and went for their weapons.

"He does not have a social security number," gasped the captain. The medic started writing. "What are you doing now?" demanded the captain.

"I'm writing 'unable to obtain' as required by EMS command, sir."

The captain's chest was tightening. The president was sweating profusely. The Secret Service still had their hands on their weapons.

"Get to the important stuff," the captain demanded. "See this patch?" the captain asked, pointing to his left shoulder. "I'm a paramedic. I know what needs to be done, so do it, now!" he hissed between gasps.

The medic looked at the captain and pointed to the *correct shoulder* sporting the medic patch.

"Sir, I know you wear the patch. But honestly, you are a book medic. You never did any time in the streets to earn it."

The neck veins stood at attention on the captain's neck. His face was flushed with rage. Sweat was soaking his white, large orange-spotted shirt. Even this MetroCare cowboy recognized pre-respiratory arrest when he was standing in front of it.

"Okay," the medic said, turning to the president, "Sir, can I please have a driver's license or Medicare card with your name, date of birth, and home address?"

The captain lunged for the medic's throat. He was intercepted by the two agents and thrown against the wall.

"He is not from this fuckin' country, you idiot!" the captain screamed.

"Yo, dude. Check yourself. You would be the first to write me up and send me to the Dragon Lady in BITS on charges if I didn't get this information. Remember sir, the fire department does not care about patient care. They are concerned with being able to bill and make money." He looked at his female partner who was beaming at him. "Besides, you are a civilian, just like me. Thus, you can't give me a direct order in that tone. Only a military officer can give a direct order."

The female medic hooked up the EKG machine to look at the president's heart. "Anybody want a printout?" she asked.

"Yes," said a tall, thin gentleman in a gray suit.

"Excuse me, who are you in relation to the patient?"

"I'm the president's doctor."

"Okay, while I do this I want you to read this Non-Solicited Medical Intervention Protocol Card."

The captain banged his head against the wall. As the medic squat down to get a copy of the EKG, there was a loud ripping sound. Perhaps it could be equated to the separation of the continental shelf, as her pants ripped at the seam before she stood up, printout in hand.

"What is all this interference on the sheet?" asked the doctor.

"I don't know. All the medics have been complaining about it but Physio Control keeps saying there is no problem with the Lifepak 12."

"How can you read it?" the doctor asked.

"We can't. I was kind of hoping you could."

Bending over the drug bag, the medic continued. "I'll start the IV."

The sight was too much for even the hardiest warrior or doctor.

"Oh no, you won't," said the president's doctor. "Only oxygen!"

The Secret Service officer was heard to mutter, "Wise choice."

After the president was packaged with the oxygen, they proceeded to the ambulance. Security was heavy as they wheeled the president out to the unit. The backdoor was opened and it was decided the stretcher with the patient could not fit in because of all the HAZMAT gear. While the crew started storing equipment, the security force got more anxious.

Just then the medic unit from Bellevue pulled in. Once again the captain took charge.

"Okay, I want you to get out your stretcher and take this patient into your ambulance," he bellowed.

"Why? They started treating. They should transport. We are always doing someone else's jobs," uttered the beastly, overweight Compensation Queen. Her last compensation case was a rule-out THA, that's Traumatic Hamburger Acquisition. Someone walked by with a hamburger and she snapped her neck following the scent. She also had three kids, one of each.

It seems she has always had a problem with authority figures. "You will do as you are told. And wipe the spaghetti sauce from your mouth!"

This didn't sit too well. But she did do as she was told and wiped her mouth with a uniform sleeve.

The captain, seething, said, "I'm the captain. Do it."

After the president was in the back of the bus, an argument broke out over who was allowed to ride.

"Hey, she is no family member," the beast bellowed, overflowing in the captain's chair, holding a Diet Coke.

"She is part of his government and goes," the captain said, slamming the side door, seeing a New York Jets Football sticker in the window.

"That's unauthorized," he yelled, as the motorcade took off for the hospital.

Choking from the diesel fumes, he approached the HAZMAT medics, who were standing outside their vehicle. It was happening to EMS. With their sellout to Fire God, and the destruction of the best EMS Academy, things were on a downhill roll. I recalled Galatians 6:7 ". . . Whatsoever a man soweth, that shall he reap." A thank you goes to all EMS civilian chiefs for a remarkable harvest of ineptness.

One morning, I was driving to work down FDR Drive, heading toward Bellevue. I had been enjoying the morning, when a car cut me off at the Thirty-fourth Street exit. As I pulled up to the car at the first light and yelled, the guy gave me the finger. Thus responding to his invitation, I cut off the car and got out.

A police sector observing the incident decided to get involved, since they saw I was in uniform. A plump individual from an Asian country, not noted for their *love of America*, told the cops they couldn't do anything to him. He was driving a car with diplomatic plates and went so far as to curse out the officers.

Continuing to taunt the cops, "Why don't you get back in your car and get out of here," he yelled. "I don't have to pay attention to your laws. You can't touch me."

I had enough. As the abusive guest continued to curse the cops and ridicule America, I spun around and nailed him twice. Onto the hood and then onto the ground went the guest.

"They can't do anything, but I sure as hell can, asshole."

"I want him arrested for assaulting me," the bloodied, irate guest screamed.

"Sorry, we can't do anything, remember?" they said, looking at the medic and smiling as they got in their car.

"Besides, we didn't see anything." I drove into Bellevue to ice my hand and the cops went for coffee. Yeah, EMS and PD work well together.

It was a gloomy night in the South Bronx. I looked at my watch. It was 1:45 A.M.. The overcast clouds hung low, emitting a cold drizzle. We sat at 149th Street and Southern Boulevard next to the twenty-four-hour White Castle Hamburger joint. The mist created a haunting world, as the diesel engine hummed, sending its polluted toxins from the exhaust pipe. I shut off the engine to hear the sound of the raindrops splattering and then slithering down the windshield.

The streets were empty except for the garbage. Papers, beer bottles, and cans littered the streets. White Castle was awash in harsh light, acting as a magnet for all sorts of street vermin.

From the bus I could see the garbage cans and the plastic bags moving in the dumpsters behind the facility. As I popped on the lights, one rat the size of a cat attacked a smaller one who had invaded its dining area. I got out, stepping on a used syringe in a foul-smelling puddle of water. Zippering my jacket, I walked inside for a coffee.

Two short, overweight Hispanic women were talking and eating. One had more hair on her chin than I had under my arms. With a hamburger in her mouth and the white cream from the shake on the pronounced mustache, she yelled in Spanish at the children. Three kids, ranging in age from four to six, played on the cold tile floor. In the other corner sat a black male who looked about sixty. He was thin, with disheveled gray hair, stubble beard, and mustache. A long, black, worn coat stretched to the floor. With weary eyes, he stared emptily into his soup. He worked the spoon, slowly stirring the hot soup, probably a donation of the generous manager.

A young Hispanic man with several young girls had walked in ahead of me. The girls ranged in age from twelve to twenty. He evidently was their "man" as evidenced by his stoic mannerisms and their dress. He was a poor imitation of Steven Seagal, but so long as he was happy, I was happy. The girls giggled and smiled.

The guy looked at me and said, "Want to have some fun tonight, paramedic? I can make you and your partner a good deal."

I liked this guy. He realized I was a paramedic and not an ambulance man. I looked at his assortment of goodies as one of the girls showed me two of her beautiful, succulent assets. They formed a circle around me and I felt one run her small hand up my crotch. Looking at her and listening to an alluring voice, I knew this girl could raise anyone's spirit.

I gently reached down and took her hand, bowed and kissed it. Looking at him I said, "Thanks, but I need the coffee to keep me up tonight."

The girl who had reached for me chimed, "But Poppy, you felt very up and alive to me." We all laughed and the girls got back in line.

As we waited, several blacks came in with their boom box wailing its rap. I had observed them exiting a beautiful, white Lexus with cream-white, dark tinted windows, gold rims. The crew wore baggy pants with oversized football jerseys, bandannas, and lots of gold. I could tell these guys were trouble. My buddy, the pimp, gave a look as two started to rap with two of his girls. The girls looked at their man and tried to ignore the interest.

"Yo bitch. You too good for me?" snapped one man, about seventeen. I stood there, thinking this was going to be a long night.

"This Spanish bitch thinks she's too good for a nigger like me," he said, as he went to grab her arm. I was starting to not like this guy. The girl was directly in front of me so I easily deflected his arm.

"Yo am-bu-lance man." He pulled away, straightening his dungaree jacket. I was, definitely, not liking him now. The gang curled around him like a snake about to strike.

"You think you bad, old man?" I guess he spotted my gray hair. I let him continue.

"You think you my father?" There was a pause.

"Shit." He went to grab the girl's neck. I intercepted his arm, throwing him off balance.

"Mother fucker!" he yelled. This time he went to lunge for me, but stopped. I stood ready for him.

"Your mother is a ho, white boy," he screamed. This young man must have had a rough day, because he certainly wasn't showing any manners, nor handling the stress well.

Realizing I had the dickhead, I said, "You are right about my mother." This stopped everyone. "But at least I know who my father is."

The old, homeless guy sitting at a table put down his soup spoon and smiled. The punk postured and jumped around while I stood watching him. Finally he stopped and looked at me.

"Don't even think about it," I said, adding, "Boy." His neck veins were popping. "I suggest you get back into your nice car and ride away from here."

"Or what, bitch?" another one chimed in.

"Or this bitch is going to kick all your motherfuckin' asses, fuck up your car, and then arrest you. Oh, and that's just for starters," I said in a calm, matter-of-fact tone. This rattled these guys, thank God.

"We outta here," said the first problem child as he went to grab a girl. I grabbed his wrist. The girl flinched. He looked at me and let go.

"You are a dead man," he screamed.

"Yeah, yeah," I said.

"Yo, nigger," the pimp said, "Enough."

"Hey, fuck you," the kid said.

The pimp opened his leather raincoat to show the Mach 10 automatic weapon under his arm. "Out now."

They cursed and left. I knew I liked this guy.

I climbed back into the vehicle with the coffee and Danish. My partner looked up from his slumber.

"You were gone for a while."

"Yeah, you know how slow these people move, filling orders. Here's a coffee and Danish when you're ready." He stretched and sat up. In typical EMS fashion, we no sooner had a bite of the Danish and a mouthful of coffee than the dispatcher called.

The job was on 149th Street and came in as an "Altered Mental Status" which was changed to an "Unconscious." As I turned the unit around, I saw the Basic unit and ELI (Emergency Locator Indicator), or fire truck merging, on the call. We offloaded our equipment and started toward a locked iron gate. Before we could gain entrance, a fireman broke the gate with his tool and said, "If you need us to break in the door, give us a call." He laughed and left.

The gate was locked as a security measure. To merely destroy property for no reason, then to laugh about it, did not sit well with any of us. It would not happen in influential Manhattan. To me it was just an act of disdain for these people, unnecessary and uncalled for. It would be different if we did not have a callback, or buzzers, or if the place was on fire.

We trudged up the narrow staircase. After three flights, we entered a cluttered apartment. A forty-five-year-old Hispanic male lay on the bed.

He had black, curly hair with a mustache. His frame was endomorphic with a fat beer belly.

The Dance of Life started when we pulled up and continued as the EMTs attempted to get vital signs and place oxygen on the patient. The patient's skin and his black dungarees were soaking wet. To his side, dressed in next to nothing, was a female in her twenties who spoke only Spanish. Diminutive in size, with shoulder-length black hair set against olive skin, she wore gold loop earrings that hung from her ears. She had a thin neck and slender body. Wringing her hands as she spoke, large black eyes darted, hoping for a good sign.

One EMT, trying not to laugh, translated, as the dance continued. The gentleman, her friend/husband, had returned from a trip to the Dominican Republic earlier in the day. After dinner and several drinks in the cramped apartment they retired to the bed, where they were making love.

Her last act was to slide down his body and start sucking his penis. As she worked him he screamed, "My head." The girl smiled, thinking it was a compliment to her nimbleness and expertise working the head of his penis. She wanted to give him a session of galactic proportions he would never forget. He stopped grabbing her head as she feverishly increased the tempo and suction. With succulent tongue wrapping around the shaft and head, her sole wish was to bring him ecstasy. He was now moaning and grabbing his head. She knew she had never felt him shake or moan like this. With a final scream, he exploded with the fury of an atomic bomb into her small mouth before collapsing. For her part, she loved him and continued to work on him swallowing the more-than-usual load of his love.

Slowly, proudly, she slid up to hold him. This was the best she had ever been. Indeed she wanted to blow his mind in pure pleasure.

It was then, only then, she noticed that something was wrong. He just lay there, limp at both ends, holding his forehead. No type of arousal worked. At first she thought he was teasing her. After her final attempt to rouse him, it dawned on her the situation was not good. She dressed him in white boxers with red hearts, then his black dungarees. With this completed, she got a large pot of cold water and dumped it on him. Don't even ask about that move. Convinced he was not faking, she made a frantic call to 911.

His blood pressure and respiration were fine, as were his pupils. We started an IV and ran the Altered Mental Status Protocol giving him thiamine (vitamin B1, which acts as an important protein to get the glucose into the cell), Dextrose (a special type of sugar, which is energy for the cells), and Narcan (a medicine that competes with and blocks opiate receptor sites, thus canceling the effect of an opiate), with no change. We packed him into the chair for the three-floor, nonstop carry down.

I put the drug bag on my back as I carried the lower part of the chair. The patient went into a fast seizure; his extremities stiffened. We were between the second and third floor on a very narrow staircase, with nowhere to put him down. His legs jutted out, kicking me in the face. His arms struck against the walls. I had one EMT holding the top of the chair. I was on the bottom, and the other two guys in single file behind him. Then I could smell the shit as his bowels let go and he urinated on himself and me.

That song "Nowhere to Run, Nowhere to Hide" sounded in my head as the urine ran down the chair and my arm.

"Fuck," I yelled, as I looked up at the terrified EMT. "Let's get him the fuck out of here!" We battled down the stairs. This guy was doing his imitation of Tom Cruise in *Mission Impossible,* with arms and legs outstretched stiff. I felt like it would be mission impossible to save him.

Downstairs, we got him into the bus and reevaluated him. His condition had gone from SNAFU (Situation Normal All Fucked Up) to TARFU (Things Are Really Fucked Up). The Dance of Life continued as one EMT hopped in the front of our bus, calling ahead to Lincoln Hospital for a standby. We noticed that his vitals were holding, but his respirations were decreasing and one pupil was blown, dilated. My partner said, "He needs to be intubated."

This night, I was working with a new medic. He made a keen observation, but didn't move on it. I sat on the floor of a bouncing, rocking bus, driving streets that would make Sarajevo, Beirut, or Northern Ireland proud, attempting to intubate. With some help, I got the guy tubed, seeing the misting on the tube as my partner listened and said he couldn't hear the tube. We needed to listen in each lung field and the stomach to make sure we heard it only in the lung fields, a whoosh of air.

"Jim, I can't hear it. You are not in," he said in a panic.

"Like hell I'm not, I had visual! Look at the fuckin' misting. I'm in."

"Jim, please. Take it out. We'll bag him." I hate a whiner, but I love it when they use the term "we." As I have learned that means, "Schrang." I did something I had never done. I extubated (removed the tube) and used only the BVM on the patient. Within a heartbeat, we pulled into the hospital. We ran into the crash room to the waiting doctors.

"Why isn't he tubed?" asked a doctor.

"I had him tubed, saw the mist, but my partner said I wasn't in. He couldn't hear the lungs," I said.

"What? If you have the mist, you have the tube," the doctor said, as he got set to drop a tube.

"Yeah, I know that. You know that. And I'm hoping now my partner knows that," I retorted. The tube went in.

"Good tube," said the doctor.

"Hey, I can't hear anything," said the nurse, listening for lung sounds.

"What? It's a good tube, I saw the chords and I see the misting," said the frustrated doctor.

"What's his oxygen sat?" (Oxygen saturation is how much oxygen the red blood cells are carrying. Below 95 percent means trouble.)

"He's at forty," said another doctor.

"How about now?" the doctor asked, as he hyperventilated the patient.

"Forty-eight" said the startled nurse.

"What the hell is going on here?" the doctor wondered aloud.

"A classic case of VQ Mismatch, I'd say," I uttered. That is when you have ventilation, but no oxygenation. Think of it as something is blocking out the oxygen from getting to the target tissues.

"Right on that, but why?" pondered the doctor, now drawing a crowd of emergency staff. As he ordered a chest x-ray I heard a little voice singing, "Knock, Knock, Knocking on Heaven's Door."

At that point, the job and this guy's life had just gone from TARFU (Things Are Really Fucked Up) to FUBAR (Fucked Up Beyond All Repair). We got the x-rays and the doctor muttered, "Holy shit!" In front of us was a gigantic embolism blocking the pulmonary artery. This artery carries the bad blood to the lungs where the bad air is exchanged for the good air. Thus, we had ventilation, but not oxygenation.

"So, let's recap this really cool job," I said to the doctor.

"The guy has an orgasm. At the moment he blows his load at one end, he literally blows his mind at the other, with a bleed on the brain. Next, as if that isn't bad enough, a blood clot breaks free and lodges so he is no longer getting adequate oxygenation."

"The classic VQ Mismatch," the doctor said.

"Sucks to be him," said one of the EMTs. .

"No," I said "sucks to be the girl. He's happy. She sure succeeded in literally blowing his mind. But she will have to go through life knowing she has lethal lips." At this point the whole staff was hysterically laughing.

"By the way, what's her name and number?" the other EMT asked.

Paramedics James "Bubba" Fallar and Guy Grillo were dispatched to a "Cardiac Arrest" in the street. The unit pulled up and Bubba jumped into action. He ran to the side compartment, opened it, grabbed the drug bag and, like a Cowboy quarterback, passed it on to Grillo. Grillo rapidly pulled the bag toward himself like he just received a handoff. He moved through the nosy civilians to get to the patient. Bubba, who will never be known as either a quarterback or Radio City Hall dancer, got his ankle caught in the concrete. All of a sudden there was a crack, then a scream, as Bubba crashed backward. Luckily, at his height, he didn't have too far to fall. As cops ran to help him, he yelled, "Don't worry about me. Get to the patient." As it turned out, the patient was dead.

There were times when even Bubba couldn't get in the way of a save. One moment was when Mirela met me at Bellevue after work. She was a young lady I had brought home with me from Bosnia. We were scheduled to go to the Big Apple Circus, which was playing on the upper West Side of Manhattan near the Lincoln Center for the Performing Arts. She showed up late, so Bubba and his partner offered to give us a ride up to the location. En route, Bubba heard of an "Injury" nearby. He decided to buff, telling the dispatcher he was close. He figured it would get us up there sooner, and the BLS would cancel us on an "Injury." I strapped in Mirela as we went ballistic. Bubba updated me that the "Injury" was changed to a "Cardiac Arrest."

I handed my jacket and camera to Mirela, telling her to stay close. She wanted to be a reporter, so I gave her the camera all set up.

After we stopped, I grabbed the monitor, passing off the drug bag to Bubba, making sure he was on the sidewalk. A crowd had formed on Fifty-seventh Street, along with the ELI, the fire truck. They sure as hell beat us there, but were doing their usual Stare of Care, nothing else.

I yelled at Mirela to stay close, as we found a male in his sixties on his back. His wife said he passed out. We stripped him and I did a quick check with the paddles. He was in V-Fib (the heart was oscillating like Jell-O).

I yelled, "I'm clear, you're clear, everyone's clear," after charging the paddles and blasting him with 200 joules of electricity.

"No pulse," Bubba said, as he lay on the sidewalk to intubate the patient.

Once the paddles were charged, I hollered, "I'm clear, you're clear, everyone's clear," and hit him with 300 joules of electricity. Bubba's tube was good and he felt a radial pulse. His partner started a line and had it in place, as Bubba pushed the medication Lidocaine to keep the heart from acting like Jell-O again.

The Basic had arrived and helped load the patient into the ambulance. They took off for Saint Luke's Hospital, two blocks away.

As the crowd dispersed, I looked at Mirela. "Okay, Hon," I said, "how many pictures did you get?"

"Pictures?" she asked.

"Yes, pictures. A man's life was just saved. You want to be a reporter and you tell me you did not take a picture?"

Well, thanks to James "Bubba" Fallar and his partner, the patient did make it, but I do not have the photos to prove it, trust me.

It was a cold December night when we received a call for an "Unconscious." I was working with a new medic and was not feeling well, fighting the flu.

We pulled up in front of a brownstone decorated for Christmas. Each side of the block was lined with trees. We climbed the frost-covered stairs and entered the small lobby. There were two new female police officers standing over the patient. The patient looked like a forty-year-old Abe Lincoln, dressed in black.

Upon his arrival home and while trying to open his door, he had the big one (heart attack), clutched his chest, and fell against his neighbor's door. The tiny woman of eighty heard a noise and opened the door. She called 911. Some of the neighbors stood on the stairs, looking at the patient. It did not take a rocket scientist to realize the guy was dead. But out of respect for my new medic partner, I said in a low, calm voice, "Do you want to work him?"

To my horror, he bellowed, "Yes, we need the practice."

I as sure as hell did not need the practice, and let's show a little class. I literally hit him with the tube kit. Then, we began working a dead person. The two female officers thought the job was on the level, so they asked to help. There we were working this dead guy, while my partner practiced and the two female cops thought they were saving a life by giving CPR.

It was going to be one of those days.

The call went in for a backup. The EMTs showed up and looked at me. Being street veterans, they knew what I knew, but misery loves company.

"Nice hats," I remarked, since both were wearing red Christmas hats. Meanwhile, my partner and the cops were out to save this dead person. Talk about a Christmas wish. Because of the patient's size, the size of the lobby, and condition of the stairs, we opted for a metal scoop to remove him.

In the back of the EMTs' bus, I looked around at the Christmas decorations taped to the walls. The back doors were open to cool us down. Suddenly the medications we had been pushing kicked in. The guy was brain dead. His soul had departed. But the medications now had the heart in V-Fib. It was strictly a chemical reaction, the heart acting like a bowel of Jell-O. To correct this, we defibrillated with the paddles.

We had the back doors of the bus open as I defibrillated the guy. Suddenly a man, looking like a pudgy Santa Claus wearing a red vest, was at the back door. He took a puff from his curved wooden pipe. The smoke danced in a curl up past his rosy cheeks that matched his red Christmas vest. Just what I fuckin' needed. Here I am with three elves and Santa just showed up. When I thought things could get worse, they did.

"Excuse me. Excuse me." When I turned, Santa continued. "Does this man live on this block?"

I ignored him and charged the paddles again. After the next jolt, as the patient did the floppy chicken, I heard, "Excuse me. I am the block president. I demand to know if the man lives on this block." I reached over to close the doors, as we were ready to go. With this he said, "Thank you for your compassion in answering me."

"Thank you for your stupidity," I responded. With this my partner and the two other elves covered their shields and nameplates simultaneously. Guess all three didn't want to blow their chances for Christmas. For my part, I hoped the Santa would land on a minefield.

Do you think my partner had enough practice for one job? Hell, no. We went to Saint Vincent's Hospital in the bus to confirm the kill. We rolled him in. One EMT did compressions, while the other was bagging. My partner and I pushed the stretcher and stopped in front of the nurse's station. In typical Saint Vincent's fashion, the nurse looked up, then continued writing. She got up, not amused by the elf wear and asked, "Why did you bring him here?"

I looked at her and said, "Because the fuckin' Port Authority was closed!"

She turned sharply. Her white pantyhose seemed to be tight after that remark. "I don't like your attitude," she hissed and walked away.

The next nurse took her shot, "Are you ALS qualified?"

I looked at her and said, "No, we just found this shit on the corner and decided to play paramedic."

"I don't—"

Before she could finish I said, "Yeah. Yeah. You don't like my attitude. How about moving your ass and getting a doctor here." She finally got a doctor. The crew moved the patient onto one of their beds. He was still on the metal scoop. The last round of medications was still kicking in, and he went into V-Fib again.

The doctor shrieked, "We can't defibrillate him on this metal thing."

They flipped the patient off the scoop. In the process they traumatically ripped out the breathing tube. They quickly rolled him over, defibrillated him once, and pronounced, "He's dead."

I looked at my partner, asking, "What did you do?"

All too often, we forgot we were dealing with people. When I first started, I was called for a "Shooting." We pulled to the corner and saw cops on the scene. The corner was loaded with drunks and I adopted the first cop's attitude I met that night.

One guy was on the ground. I ran my hands up and down his back and chest under his shirt. Finding no blood, I took the guy to be just another drunk. They called in as "Unconscious" or "Shot" just to get a bus to pick up their drunk friend. Or Mr. Yuppie calls to get a homeless guy removed from in front of his store or apartment.

I was pissed to be stuck with another drunk, pissed the medics were called for a drunk.

"What have you got?" the medic asked.

"A fuckin' drunk."

"What do you want to do?"

"Contact sanitation," I said. Macho statement, right? Wrong. Real asshole statement. He was drunk, right? Correct. We loaded him into the back of the bus. As I started to take vital signs, he kept putting his hand inside his shorts. There was no blood.

Finally, I listened to my little voice, which was screaming by now. I closed the door and pulled his pants and shorts off. Looking around, I did not see anything, until I moved his penis to one side.

"The guy was fuckin' shot," I yelled to the medic, Don Boyce.

"Don, I fucked up. The guy was shot."

Don climbed aboard. The guy evidently had his pants pulled down. The small-caliber weapon was put next to the skin and fired. The burn cauterized the wound.

I was exhausted and had adopted the cop's attitude. There was no excuse, no matter how exhausted, to fall into this trap. I'm glad to say it never happened again.

Years later, Don was teaching and asked if he could use this experience as a lesson. Without a hesitation, I said yes. I fucked up and really could have hurt this person. I could handle the embarrassment if it helps even one medic avoid the pitfalls of the street. I'm better for the patient and having Don as a medic by my side.

I was on overtime out of Elmhurst Hospital, with a third-year doctor aboard, and got a call for a "Difficult Breather," a female forty years old.

The family had brought her from Mexico for cancer therapy. The cancer had metastasized, spread all over her body, including her brain. She had been in a nursing home, but the family wanted her to die at home. A noble thought, until it sunk in that the young woman would be dead before the sundown. On a guilt trip, they called 911.

We arrived, got the story, and placed her in the back of the bus, making her as comfortable as possible. Both of us knew she would pass on before we got to the emergency room.

En route to the hospital the doctor asked me, "Aren't you going to intubate her?" I reached over and gave the tube kit.

After she intubated the patient, she asked, "What about an IV?"

Without a word, I reached over and gave her the setup, and then I bagged the patient as we pulled into the hospital bay. My partner opened the door and looked with shock at the patient then at me. Both of us had enough experience to know better. Later, as I was filling out the paperwork, the young doctor came over to me.

"Why weren't you going to do anything? I thought you are supposed to work to save lives?" she asked, honestly seeking an answer.

"Please follow me, doctor," as we walked to the crash room. Inside, we saw a staff running around, working on the terminal patient. A machine breathed for her since she would never breathe on her own again. The patient was naked on a sterile metal table under stark light. She was poked and prodded, and all sorts of needles with wires were attached to her. Her blood was on the floor. Some of the older doctors talked and joked with the newer medical students, who were taking notes.

"What do you see, doctor?"

"I see them working to save a life," she responded.

"Look again," I said softly. "She is terminal. Are they giving her any type of respect? They are joking, playing, if you will. In their heart they know she will not recover. Yet they prolong her agony for two reasons. One, so they can play, second, out of fear of their own mortality. This is a person, doctor, not a cancer case, broken femur, or gallbladder. This is a person, a living soul."

One doctor asked the other, "What have you got?"

"A cancer job."

I looked at the female doctor and continued, "She is not a cancer job, a broken leg, or a heart attack. She is a person. You spoke of saving lives. If it was meant sarcastically, how dare you. Since I don't believe you meant it that way, I'll say this. Both my partner and I and those EMS people," I pointed to a group of EMTs and medics at different stages of triage with patients, "any of those EMS people will fight like hell for the living. But they believe in the quality of life, not quantity of days, hours, or years. We have learned this truth through years of dealing with patients, seeing them as people. Not only hearing them, but *listening to* them." He walked away to continue his paperwork.

Later, as we stood together at the unit, the young doctor came over.

"Hey guys, I could use a cup of coffee. Let's go to Starbucks."

"Typical female, always the expensive type," I said. We all laughed.

"No, this is on me as well as dinner. You taught me a lesson they never teach us in medical school. After you left me standing there, I was scared. I thought, *what if I had not learned this today? It might have taken me years to learn it. God, I became a doctor to help. I could have spent years pushing medications, learning, but never really knowing.*"

We accepted the coffee offer, but not dinner. We had found a new friend but, more importantly, witnessed the birth of a healer.

Great Grandmother Moon was a beautiful, white ball, sinking beyond the horizon of the concrete buildings. We had coffee on a side street in Washington Heights in upper Manhattan. This area is known to us as Dominican Land because of the large population of hardworking immigrants and sensual Dominican girls. I could feel the warmth of the sun as I sat with my partner in the cramped unit. It was a peaceful morning. The city was still shaking the slumber from its eyes. Small bodegas and bagel shops put on fresh coffee for the Saturday night party crowd returning home.

The tranquility was broken as a medic unit received a "Shooting." I listened with one ear, not particularly interested one way or the other. After the unit was on the scene, they reported that they had a female shot and needed a surgical standby at Harlem Hospital. The victim stated that there was at least one more person shot. The crew suggested to the dispatcher that another unit respond while they left the scene. We volunteered.

We pulled up to the location overlooking Highbridge Park, just as the other unit pulled away with its critically shot patient. One police officer approached us, as an EMS patrol boss, Lieutenant Pam Hehn, pulled up.

Pam was a good boss and it was a pleasure to see her. The officer said they had found one other victim, an 83 (10-83 means dead). I asked if there were any other victims and he said he had no idea. I suggested that my partner remain with the bus. It wasn't clear how many people were shot and perhaps another victim would make it to the bus, escaping through the woods. Also, my partner had a good portion of his breakfast uneaten. The cop said I was going down to pronounce a "dead person."

Through the years, I've been on more than one job where the cop has declared the patient dead when we, EMS people, raised that person from the dead. Sometimes we even literally walked the dead person to the bus in front of the startled cop. The good lieutenant grabbed the oxygen bag as I pulled out the trauma bag and followed the cop.

Once off the road, we entered the pristine tree line. My boots kicked up some dust, as we walked a dirt trail heading deeper into the park. The sun's warmth had yet to reach the ground foliage, which still had glorious pearls of dew dripping from its lush leaves. The trunks of the trees bore scars from carved messages, destroying the protective bark. Garbage from indifferent parkgoers littered the trail. The deeper into the forest we traveled, the further we left humans and civilization behind. A blue jay sang, as little animals moved under the foliage. A small deer looked at the trespassers.

The trauma bag cut deep into my shoulder, as sweat soaked the collar of my shirt. We walked in silence. Each of us was lost in our own thoughts as we went deeper into this cathedral of nature. The air felt cool, clean, and energized. Each of us was reverently afraid to utter a word and break the holy magical moment of Mother Earth's cathedral.

We entered a clearing, twenty by thirty feet. The victim was under a tree. I dropped the bag and put on my blue gloves. The girl appeared to be in her twenties. She was naked. Her legs were spread, her arms outstretched.

I observed a small-caliber hole with an entry, no exit hole, to the right side of her head. A thin stream of dried blood stained her hair. Thick, black eyelashes encased her brown eyes. They were open and had a shocked look. Her mouth was open, as if uttering "Why?" Her lifeless, nude body was small in frame. Her complexion was a light brown, likely Hispanic. Her black hair was short. There were no scars or track marks on her body; her skin had been well maintained.

I squatted next to the body, going through the motions of feeling for a pulse, then saw it. Her right hand, in a death grip, held a cheap, red, white, and blue beaded bracelet. In the sacred silence of Mother Nature's cathedral, this girl died violently. Alone, she lay upon the soft forest floor of pine needles, looking with empty eyes toward the rising sun. The sun's rays caressed her body, turning it a rich golden texture. On the way back, we saw portions of clothing thrown in disarray. The lieutenant and I walked back to our vehicles in silence.

Later, I learned that both victims had enjoyed the excitement of the fast life. Finding hustling boring, they robbed drug dealers' houses.

Now caught, they were herded down the trail in the early morning light, like two lost sheep to the slaughter. The petrified girls were shoved, smacked, threatened and ordered to strip as they walked. Once at the clearing they were ordered to remove the rest of their clothing and jewelry. Somehow the smaller, younger one hid the bracelet. The morning chill silently cut through their bodies as they stood together, not knowing their fate. The trees loomed like gigantic buttresses around them, supporting an endless crystal-clear blue sky of unlimited possibilities above them. The dirt under their feet, still cool and moist from the evening mist, had a nurturing energy neither girl had ever known. Their senses were on overdrive. The forest smelled clean, invigorating.

The dealer opened a small bottle and sniffed in its contents, as his friend finished his beer. Without a word, the older, black female—the surviving girl—was made to kneel. Her captor held a nine-millimeter Berretta in his right hand. Understanding, she reached up, opening his belt and pants. After lowering his pants and shorts to his ankles, she opened her mouth and started to suck him. The younger girl watched before being abruptly pulled by her hair to an area about fifteen feet away. While the older girl was giving a blowjob, she saw her friend being enjoyed. The younger girl gagged as her head was violently forced back and forth. Pants and shorts at his ankles, the other man's pale flat backside and stringbean legs looked almost funny to her.

He was cursing the petite girl. The black girl was shocked by the violence of the act being forced upon the smaller friend. It was then she saw the beaded bracelet. How strange, she thought, that her friend would hold on to something that cheap, that worthless. She had taken it from her mother, a mother she hated. It was a gift given to her as a baby by a now dead father.

They only made eye contact once as the girl was violently shoved onto her back. Brown eyes were filled with terror and confusion. The sight of her distraught, naked friend sent a foreboding chill down her spine. She heard the dealer's order to spread. As the black girl continued to suck the male, bringing him closer to an orgasm, she watched the dealer. He cruelly entered her friend and began pumping in a brutal frenzy. There was a childlike whimper. Her friend's legs and arms spread outstretched, obediently. Only the grunting and cursing of the dealer could now be heard. Then the silence of the morning was broken as he moaned, collapsing onto the petite spread-eagled friend.

Suddenly, she felt the cold steel of the Berretta as it rested on her shoulder. Her captor held the back of her head lightly, as he watched the dealer. The world was silent. Then there was an ear-splitting explosion. It startled both her and captor, who ejaculated uncontrollably into her mouth. The dealer slowly turned, while still in her lifeless friend. Her friend's head was thrust upward, mouth open, silent. He fiendishly looked at the black girl, her mouth covered in sperm, still holding her captor's penis in her now trembling hand. The horror hit her as a sinister smile appeared on his crazed face.

The girl reacted, quickly pushing her captor off balance, bolting, screaming hysterically, running for her life, entering the tree line. Shots were fired in rapid succession, cracking as they passed her head. Birds shrieked in terror as the sacred silence was shattered. Tree bark exploded, as round after round found a mark. Suddenly slammed by a tremendous force, she felt two rounds crash into her back and arm. Uncontrollably tumbling through thick foliage, she finally came to a violent stop in a depression. In a drunken, drug-induced rage, the two men, cursing, blindly fired, emptying their weapons into the woods at the edge of the clearing. Trying to control her breathing, she lay there waiting, praying. Now the full impact of witnessing her friend murdered in cold blood hit. Burying her face in the soft, moist earth to smother the sobs, she let her tears form puddles before being absorbed into the ground, just as people are when death comes and the body decays back into the ground.

Fighting to regain control of her breathing, she felt the physical pain become excruciating. Her right arm was numb, though she could feel the shattered bone. Again, breathing was becoming a problem as her chest felt on fire. Realizing to survive she would have to move, now, slowly the girl crawled around the side of the hill, moving to the south of the clearing. Finally, not hearing her captors, she clawed her way up the hill. After what seemed like hours, she got to the road, and a phone, calling 911. EMS was first on the scene.

There were times when the Street Saints of Compassion received help from people. All too often the situation was critical. We were focused on the patient and never got the chance to say thank you. Sometimes, these people faded into the crowd and became as invisible as the Street Saints. Usually, they were adults. Sometimes, they were remarkably gifted younger people.

Below is the story of one such heroine who saw the need and assisted in saving her grandmother's life.

Angelo Morales and I received a call for an "Asthma Critical." The computer-generated information stated that the patient was a fifty-five-year-old female, who was having an attack. The classification was critical asthma because she had been intubated twice before.

We pulled up to the house on the dark street. The fresh fallen snow was dirty from the pollution. As we got out of the bus, the cold, wet wind cut into us unmercifully.

It would be nice if someone in the fire department would design foul-weather gear for us, I thought. We proceeded to retrieve our equipment and headed toward the dilapidated abode. We entered the dimly lit dwelling. The foul smell was what first hit us. The smell came from the poor sanitation system in the two-story house. We were directed into the starkly lit kitchen that was filthy with cigarette butts and dust. We observed a short, plump Hispanic woman, our patient. She grasped the refrigerator for balance and used a home nebulizer, without relief.

Angelo switched her to our nebulizer and oxygen bottle. I listened to her lungs. She was hardly moving any air. The daughter on the scene was not much help. She didn't grasp how critical her mother was.

Angelo and I knew that if we did not act fast, the patient would crash. She would go into respiratory arrest, then cardiac arrest. The survival rate at that point would be slim to none. South Bronx was the asthma capital and another patient was about to die. The Dance of Life started as we loaded her into the stair chair. She was becoming combative due to hypoxia. Her respiratory system was constricting, becoming clogged with mucus, decreasing her ability to exchange gases. She had the "thousand-yard stare" that veterans and paramedics know too well. Her accessory muscles were trying to help her breathe, but it was a losing battle.

I grabbed the equipment and ran to the bus. I returned to help Angelo. He already had her strapped into the stair chair. We dragged and carried this woman through the filthy snow to the back of the bus. I climbed up and we lifted her into the back. We moved her onto the stretcher, cursing as we tried to collapse the stuck chair in the narrow confines of the ambulance.

We encouraged her to concentrate on breathing. Angelo was getting the archaic, twelve-watt radio out to call telemetry for orders.

A family member, a young girl, had climbed on board for the trip to the hospital. I was having about as much luck getting IV access as the patient was having breathing. Her hands were soaked, as they started slipping from my gloved hands. I removed my blue gloves, trying to get a better grip.

"Angelo. She's going to crash," I said and asked the young girl to step out the back for a minute. I promised her that we would not leave without her. As she stepped from the back, the woman's eyes rolled into her head, and she went into respiratory arrest. I lowered her head and Angelo set up to intubate her.

"Think it's time for a backup?" he asked. I love when he asks such understated questions.

"I can do that," I said, almost smiling, as I got rid of the catheter I was holding. "Two Six Will. Two Six Will," I said into the portable, moving around the back of the bus for better reception.

"Two Six William," the dispatcher responded.

"Two Six Will. I need EMTs. We have a respiratory arrest."

I always specify EMTs so they do not send the firefighters. The EMTs have more knowledge and will be more help. As we continued the Dance of Life, we heard the dispatcher assign us a backup. The backup was telling the dispatcher that there were closer units to us than they were.

The response was, "You are the first recommended." Gee, how I missed the days of Mickey and her style of dispatching. She knew her units, would listen, and then make a decision. Today, in the world of the Fire God, the control freaks changed the rules. Dispatchers do not make such decisions. They must go by what the computer says. I was going to get on the radio and tell the dispatcher to listen to the unit, but we were busy. Angelo got the tube and I double checked for placement. It was a good tube.

At this point, we realized the backup was going to be a while getting to us, and we needed more hands. I kicked open the back door and called the girl to get into the bus. Once inside, she stood before us, taking in the scene. Her grandmother was blue. A tube was projecting out her mouth and the one medic was squeezing a bag attached to it. There was no response from the woman. Her lifeless body was slumping off the stretcher. Blood was slowly dripping from an IV attempt onto the floor.

I asked, "Do you want to help?"

Without hesitation, she replied firmly, "Yes."

"Fine, get your jacket off. Now put these on," I said, handing her a pair of blue gloves. "You are going to breathe for grandma until we can get her to breathe on her own." I had her straddle the patient and showed her how to breathe for the patient using the BVM. As the little heroine kept her grandmother alive by breathing for her, Angelo and I continued our work. The patient received some medications down the tube and we finally got IV access in her short, fat neck. In the distance, I could hear the cavalry coming.

As I have so often stated, paramedics save patients and good EMTs save paramedics. It is truly a team effort, this Dance of Life. This young lady was a viable team member in the dance.

I asked her name. Straddling her grandmother and keeping her alive with the breath of life, she replied, "Yasnery."

Her shoulder-length hair cascaded down in front of her shoulders. Piercing, vibrant eyes observed everything. It was only then I realized how young she appeared. I heard the backup outside and yelled to them. As they climbed aboard, they thought we had a medical student with us.

"Who are you?" one of the EMTs asked. Looking over her shoulder, still breathing for the grandmother, she replied.

"That's my grandmother." Both EMTs looked in amazement.

"How old are you?" one asked.

"I'm thirteen."

One of the EMTs took her to the front of the bus, but not before hugging her. His partner took over breathing for the patient. The dance continued. The woman, now intubated, with IV access attained, and medications on board, started to projectile vomit. "Roll her on her side," I said.

"I'll get the suction going," said Angelo. With one EMT and me holding the patient on her side, she continued to vomit and Angelo suctioned. For what seemed an eternity, it seemed he was losing the battle as wave after wave of vomit violently splashed onto the floor. The stench in the back was unbelievable. Finally, she stopped, and we laid her back. I rechecked the tube placement. It was still good. A notification was made to Jacobi Hospital. Of course, it is not Bellevue, or even Lincoln, but I was praying for a miracle.

As Angelo and I worked on the woman, I sent Reiki energy (Ancient form of Japanese energy healing) to her. Suddenly, she opened her eyes.

Angelo spoke to her in Spanish and she responded. The EMTs drove, and soon we were safely there. We brought the patient to the crash area.

Later I walked out to Yasnery, who was with one of the EMTs.

"Listen, Hon, I have to tell you how very proud I am of you. If I had a daughter, I would want her to be just like you. Do you know where McDonald's is in this hospital?"

"Yes," she responded. I reached in my pocket and pulled out some money.

"I want you to get something to eat," I told her as we walked. "Wait there for me, okay?" She promised and proceeded down the hall. I gave my report.

"Thanks, Jim," I heard the doctor say.

"You do not remember me, do you?" he asked.

"No, sir, I'm sorry," I replied.

"Well, I was a new doctor at Bellevue about eight years ago. I remember you," he said with a smile. Gee, another miracle.

Later, I went back to get Yasnery. The registrar wanted to meet her. It is not too often we meet people of Yasnery's character and courage. As I approached, she was sitting alone, sipping a soda.

"Did you eat?"

"No, I wasn't too hungry," she said softly.

"Well, let's you and me take a walk. The registrar needs some information perhaps you can give her." She stood up, placing the soda container in the garbage can. I looked at this courageously gifted miracle. We approached the door and I opened it for her.

"Thank you," she whispered.

"What do you want to be when you grow up?" I asked.

"An actress," she said in a wistful way. Even at her tender age, she realized not too many dreams come true, living in South Bronx. There were remarkable stories of success. But these were the minority, not majority of cases. In my experience with the people of the South Bronx, I saw a fertile land of untapped talent and flourishing dreams.

"Well, you sure won the Academy Award today. You were so in control and professional, the EMTs thought you were a medical student," I said, as I saw a slight smile. As we started walking down the long stark hallway, I put my arm around this uncut diamond, this true wonder, Yasnery.

Some of the most interesting moments came with people on a different frequency, shall we say. Instead of calling someone an EDP, I prefer FMD (Frequency Modulated Disease).

We are all energy. Energy vibrates at different frequencies. This EDP was operating on a different frequency from us as he sat talking to someone, someone we couldn't see. *Is he crazy? Maybe, or is he actually conversing?*

The junkies were another interesting group, not the little white girl from the upper middle-class suburb in Connecticut, but the everyday hard user.

A paramedic unit pulled up to an "Unconscious" call. It was dusk, so the older paramedic appreciated the ELI fire truck lights marking the location. As usual, they were standing around, looking like a group of penguins. As the medic approached, he got the usual, "Oh, we just pulled up."

Of course, they got the usual from the older medic, "Thanks, pickup, and have a safe tour."

He made contact with the unconscious patient along with his frantic friends. Thus the Dance of Life began. His partner started to bag the patient.

"What is he on?" asked the medic, as if he didn't know.

"Heroin," replied the concerned citizen.

Both medics noticed the engine company hanging around.

"You guys going to be okay?" the fire officer asked.

"Yeah, thanks for asking." Both medics realized the firemen wanted to see what was about to happen.

"We gave him a home remedy and it just didn't work," said the friend, as the medic drew up the Narcan.

"What was that, my friend?" the medic inquires.

"Oh, we gave him a shot of vegetable oil."

"Into his veins?"

"Yes, but it didn't work."

Both medics heard the firemen laugh. As the medic gave the Narcan, he stated, "Of course, it didn't work. You didn't give him carrots and red beets."

They heard the fireman say, "What the hell?" Now they were really listening. The cops who knew the medics stood there, grinning.

"Is this clown on the level?" the fire officer asked the cop.

"First, he is a paramedic. Second, if you listen you may learn something. Third, if anything happens to me, I certainly want these guys to take care of me."

The patient started to regain consciousness.

The junkie said, "I can't fit a carrot and beet in the syringe. I'm not stupid."

"I know you are not. Just hear me out. Did you ever hear of a juicing machine?"

"Oh yeah. Now I understand. But why the carrot and beet?"

"Okay. First, the carrot has carotene, which is an antioxidant. It cleans up pollution in the body."

"Okay," says the thoughtful junkie. "The beet?"

"Hey buddy, just lie there and relax," the medic said to the patient, as his partner placed an oxygen mask on him.

"The beet is to increase the red blood cells."

"I've heard that," the junkie said.

In the background he heard someone say, "Thus you mix the carotene, the cleanser, with the beets, increasing the red blood cells. The mix, with the olive oil, not vegetable oil, cleans the system."

"Wow, that's great. So we don't have to call you guys?"

"Uh, not quite. It will take a while for you to mix everything, right?"

"Yeah."

"Well, during this period of time, brain cells are dying because you are not breathing, right?"

"Yeah."

"Thus you need us. However, if you drink the mix I just suggested, you won't be sick when we give you the Narcan."

"Really."

"Right. Because—"

Before he could finish, the junkie blurts out, "Because my blood will be cleaner and stronger."

"There you have it, my friend." NYC paramedics believed an informed patient and one who participates in his/her healing was a happy patient.

A medic unit sat at 110th Street and Broadway outside a bagel shop. Two students from Columbia approached the crew.

"Could you please explain to my friend that the brain heats up as you use it to think?" The one medic looked at his partner, gave him a sheepish grin and put his bagel down. His partner opened the *New York Times*, not wanting to be part of what was about to transpire.

"You are a hundred percent correct," said the medic.

"See, I told you," said the dweeb student from the prestigious college.

"But did you know there is also an easy way to increase that activity, say while studying for an exam?" asked the medic.

"Yeah. Anyone knows if you take uppers (amphetamines), they will increase your alertness," the student responded.

"Ha, but uppers cause side effects. Did you ever use Ben Gay?"

"Sure on my muscles when they are sore."

"Okay. You two seem like you are smart and won't spread this around. What happens, what do you feel?" asked the medic, knowing he was now reeling in two educated idiots.

"It gets hot," one student proclaimed proudly.

"Correct. And that means, what is happening to the cells to produce more heat?"

The other chimed in, "They are moving faster."

"Great. So what would happen if you applied it to the skull?"

"It would seep in and," then it hit them, "and increase your brain activity."

"You got it, guys," said the smiling medic. And you think these kids don't learn in college.

"Man, that's awesome. I knew I was right to ask you guys."

The other student looked. "How much and where?"

The medic went on to explain, placing large globs on the temples (sides), occipital (back), and frontal lobes above the eyes. For optimal results, sleep with it on your head. The two happy students walked away to buy Ben Gay. NYC paramedics were always happy to teach.

These are stories I could never make up in my wildest dreams. They happened every day on the streets of New York.

On this job, I met some very remarkable people, especially working in Midtown Manhattan. One such person was Attorney Barry Slotnik. I was giving "expert testimony" against his client. When it was over, his client went to the slammer for a contracted hit, along with his wife.

As I walked out, Mr. Slotnik took the time to tell me I did a great job. He did his best to rattle me on the stand. After a few barbs back and forth, the judge got into the act.

"Mr. Schrang. You will have to answer Mr. Slotnik's question."

I took a sip of water, smiled at two female jurors, asking, "Then you want me to lie?" Needless to say, Mr. Slotnik was trying to lead my testimony in a direction I would not go. In the end, I prevailed, and his client went to jail. I have to say that without a shadow of a doubt, Barry Slotnik was one of those people I liked the moment I met him, no matter the side. He was tenacious in the courtroom, but gracious outside.

It was a warm summer afternoon when I pulled into Bellevue at Twenty-sixth Street and First Avenue. Directly across the street to the south is Hunter College of Nursing. Construction crews had been on the roof, repairing it after a long cold winter. As I walked around the corner of the garage, I was almost struck by a bus driven by Paramedic James "Bubba" Fallar. His partner covered his eyes as I dove to avoid getting hit. When Bubba was behind the wheel, he was a terror. *He probably forgot the training blocks to reach the gas and brake pedal*, I thought. So, at warp factor one, he took off.

As I walked into the office, I smelled smoke and turned to see where it was coming from. The roof of the college was totally engulfed in flames. Black, putrid smoke billowed into the blue sky.

"Waa waa. Fire. Fire. Fire. Oh. Waa, For the love of humanity! Waa. Ambulances. Fire!. Fire! Send ambulances. Oh, the fire."

"Unit with an emergency. Unit, what's going on?" the startled dispatcher yelled between the pleas for humanity. As I got into the unit, I told the confused dispatcher, I would give a 10-12 (Situation Report).

Bubba had pulled up on Twenty-fifth Street. I had pulled up on Asser Levy Place. The MERV driven by EMT Dave Soto and a Basic unit followed me. Once in place, leaving the units on Twenty-third Street for best access and egress, I attempted to give my report. "Stress Free to Central."

"Central, go."

"Okay. We have a fire at Hunter College. The roof is engulfed."

Before I could finish, Navy Seal wannabe Lieutenant Paul Giblin got on the air: "Thirteen Patrol, Thirteen Patrol," he bellowed.

"Central, please tell Thirteen Patrol to stay off the air and report to my staging location," I requested.

Before the dispatcher could say anything, Giblin blubbered into the radio, "I'm in charge! I'm Thirteen patrol!" You can't help but love this guy.

The dispatcher toned him.

"Thirteen Patrol, stay off the air. Stress Free, continue." As I reiterated our staging area and resources, the flames climbed to the sky. I had set us upwind so I was not concerned, but the potential for problems was indeed high as the fire department pulled up. EMT Dave Soto and others stood next to me as I gave an update.

"Levy Command to Central with a twelve." (I had been given this designation by the dispatcher).

"Levy Command, go."

"Potential is high, and still no Boss at my location. Holding with current resources." There was a pause, and then a tremendous explosion shook us all. A propane tank on the roof ignited and took off like a rocket, sending shrapnel everywhere. I said over the roar, "Be advised we have had a positive detonation." Then I thought. They would never understand, so I said, "That's explosion." I turned and everyone that had been standing with me was gone. They were up the block behind their vehicles.

As the fire raged, the fire department went on the roof for an aggressive fight. The burned and injured were brought to the Twenty-fifth Street staging area, but they had an egress problem. I gave another twelve when Lieutenant Giblin again got on the air and told me to report to him. "I'm the boss."

"Negative," I said. "I will not leave my command or resources."

A chief came on the air and told Lieutenant Giblin to report to *my* sector. I turned and saw the chief there. "Want to take over, Boss?" I asked.

"No, you are doing fine."

Before Lieutenant Giblin got to my sector, another patrol boss showed up and I turned it over to him. Paramedic James "Bubba" Fallar made history once again with what came to be known as Bubba's Von Hindenburg 12. My hero.

Through the years I have been blessed to work with the best, including outstanding new medics. Medics will not stay, like me, because of the bullshit. The loss of medics like Justin Enzmann, Mike Markowski, and Bryan Melchionda will have a direct impact on the care the public receives. But then, the only ones who have ever been interested in patient care have been the paramedics and EMTs.

I had the pleasure of working with Bryan one day in Manhattan aboard 07Y2. We were seated at Thirty-fourth Street and Sixth Avenue across from Macy's, the world's largest department store. A call came in for a "Pedestrian Struck" at 305 West Thirty-sixth Street.

EMS dispatching, being on top of the situation, right, attempted to send a New York Hospital paramedic unit at Forty-third Street and Second Avenue to back up the Basic unit.

If EMTs John Jagoda and Alex Carrasquillo were calling, it had to be bad. I got on the air and told the dispatcher we were 10-89, closer. Reluctantly, he got around to giving it to us as we pulled up the wrong way on a one-way street.

On this nice, warm day, America's most lethal weapon struck a worker standing by his truck. The most lethal weapon we have in the American arsenal is the Oriental female driving with New Jersey plates. I'd put her up against any cab drivers in Manhattan and she will win each time for doing the unexpected.

On this particular day, the woman came out of the basement garage at warp factor five and out of control. The worker was standing next to his truck, when she traumatically amputated his lower right leg, slamming him into his truck. Police Officer Jeff Stella stated, "He was bleeding badly and his leg was off." Thinking he was doing the right thing, he used his leather belt as a tourniquet. This, of course, was the wrong thing, but I gave him credit.

When we approached, FD Rescue One was on the scene, along with a Basic unit from Bellevue. The street was pandemonium and chaos as another engine pulled up. The bystanders were trying to see the blood and gore. Couple this with the media and there was hell.

I got to the patient and saw the belt tourniquet.

"Who the fuck put that on?" I asked. The fireman from Rescue One responded, "A cop did it." "Was the blood spurting from an arterial wound?"

The fireman who had helped the Basic crew put on a multi-trauma said, "No."

I removed the damn tourniquet. In most cases of traumatic amputation, and I saw a lot in Bosnia, the wound itself will be seared, closed by the heat of the insulting mechanism of trauma. We use a tourniquet as a last resort. The tourniquet cuts the blood flow to the tissues below, so everything below the tourniquet dies. In this case, if Bellevue Hospital was hoping to do a replant, they would have nothing to work with. But there would be no replant attempt since the car had created a jagged, uneven wound.

As the crew loaded him up, I ran to the back of the BLS bus, which was open and set up. One of the firemen from Rescue One brought up the lower leg, wrapped just as it is supposed to be, and I loaded it on the bus. These guys were great. Bryan evaluated the patient as he was loaded.

Rescue One did a great job in packaging. The fire captain asked what he could do and if I needed help. The patient was thrashing in pain, so I requested one of his men ride with us. We moved toward Bellevue, picking up speed, finally going ballistic. John was up front, driving, and Alex had already called in the notification.

One crew was asked to respond to an MVA (Motor Vehicle Accident). The patrol boss on the scene requested a paramedic unit, but did not state why. As the crew pulled up, they noticed a car had run into the back of an open truck. The truck had been carrying Chinese laborers. They sat on the sidewalk without complaints of injury from the low kinetic impact. They stated that the driver of the car, a livery cab, was drunk and abusive. As one of the paramedics walked past the car, he noticed a one hundred dollar bill on the visor. When he got to the patient, a male from India, he saw the patrol boss.

The patrol boss looked like one of the characters from the Adams Family Show, Uncle Fester, short and rotund in shape. His bald head shone in the evening sunlight, along with his spanking new, white paramedic patch on his shoulder. He wanted to "play" (do some ALS, Advanced Life Support) if it was warranted.

The driver of the car stood next to the ambulance, as the paramedic approached.

"Sir, does anything hurt?"

"No."

"Okay. Don't move a moment while I get a set of vitals." The medic went to touch the patient's wrist and he pulled back cursing the medic.

"Fuck you. Don't touch me."

"Listen, we are here to help. How about if I take your blood pressure to ensure you are okay?" As the medic went to put the cuff on the obnoxious patient's arm, he tried to shove the medic. The medic stepped aside and, using the patient's forward momentum, slammed him into the side door of the bus.

"Okay, you don't want help. Fine," said the medic. "But I would suggest you allow me to clean up that nasty slash you have above your left eye from walking into the door of my ambulance." This was going nowhere. "Sir, I want to place you on the long board, okay?" After the guy cursed, the medic stood there.

The lieutenant chimed in, "Listen pal, I'm a lieutenant, his boss. You have to go on the long board and get vital signs taken."

"Fuck off."

"Try again," the lieutenant orders the medic.

"No," was the response. He turned to the medic's partner.

"Do you want to take his vital signs?"

"If my partner don't, I don't."

"Hey," said the first medic, "you're a paramedic. Why don't you take them?"

Both medics started to laugh. After a few minutes the patient was "assisted" into the back of the bus and "secured" to the long board. It seemed he did not want to do it the easy way outside. With a rapid take-down, he was "assisted." Patient care is always our utmost concern, second only to finding a good coffee location.

The patient was in the back, when the medic driving said to his partner, "Listen. Since there is a sensitivity problem here, why don't we change places? You drive, and I'll take care of him." His partner concurred, noting a twinkle in his eye and a smile on his lips.

As the medic climbed in, he called to the unwitting lieutenant who put them in this mess. "Hey, come up and give me a hand will you?"

He responded with enthusiasm envisioning starting a real IV. The first medic sat up front. The bus had a small plastic window dividing the crew from the patient compartment. Soon, it happened.

He heard the patient shouting and cursing as his partner said, "Sir, please stop fighting. I'm trying to find a vein with this fourteen gage needle." That was the largest needle we carry. More cursing continued.

As the medic looked through the window, he saw the once glistening head of the boss covered with a layer of sweat. As he too wrestled with the patient, the other medic said in a calm, monotone voice. "Sir, I have to get this IV. I intend to make sure you get everything you deserve."

"Hey, boss?" called the medic in the front. "Ever try getting a neck vein?" After numerous unsuccessful IV attempts by the boss, he decided to transport. At other times in world history it might been known as Bloodletting 101.

The medic unit hauled because the boss wanted to play after all. As the disheveled, boss left the vehicle, the medic in the back called to his partner.

"I want a standby with a surgical team at Bellevue Hospital for this man." His partner understood.

"Are you strapped in?"

"Oh, yeah." He knew what was about to transpire as the unit picked up speed, siren wailing. In the side mirror, the medic driving chuckled as he spotted the boss. He was attempting to tuck his new, blood-spattered sweatshirt into his pants. His radio fell still attached to his work belt. As he grabbed for the radio, his pants fell from his large stomach to his knees, giving the locals a great laugh.

"Cute boxer shorts. I wonder if they make them for men," chuckled the medic.

There was a life to save, so the medic's attention was turned back to the job at hand, driving. As he cut across numerous lanes of traffic, he had to lock the brakes to avoid being struck several times by America's most lethal weapon, females driving with New Jersey plates.

The screaming patient finally got to be too much. So the driver reached over and turned on the local oldies station. With "Only In America" by Jay and The Americans blasting, the medic found solitude and concentrated on driving, without distractions from the shrieking patient.

The vehicle was now at warp factor five, above ballistic, as the crew hurdled through the canyons of Manhattan. Of course, they were asking themselves the proverbial question: Why?

As the medic decelerated rapidly, loosing the kinetic energy of the run, he hung a right turn into Bellevue Hospital, past the infamous Men's Shelter. He noticed a patient he and his partner helped the previous week. The older, black gentleman was in his wheel chair and waved frantically. The bus was about thirty feet past the old man when the medic locked the brakes and threw it in reverse, sending gravel and smoke flying. Once beside of the old man, the medic turned down the radio and lowered the window.

"Pop, is everything okay?" he asked.

"Oh, I just wanted to thank you and your partner for saving my life."

"Glad we could help. But now you need to take you medicine. Okay?"

"Yeah, I will. Tell your partner I said thanks and God bless you both."

"You too, pop." He waved as the bus picked up speed. It was rare to hear a thank you from someone we helped.

As the bus approached the service road, the medic turned to avoid hitting a diamond-shaped, concrete island in the path of the vehicle. But the turning radius was bad and bam,up on the island; bam, off of the island they went, accompanied by curses from the rear. Just can't please some people. They want a fast ride to the hospital, but don't take into consideration the work of the highly trained paramedic or EMT.

Arriving in the emergency bay, the medic shut off the bus, got out, and walked through the haze of burning rubber to open the rear door. His partner, sitting serenely in the captain's chair, put down the copy of Gear, adorned with Penelope Cruz. He unbuckled his safety belt and smiled as he stepped out.

"Nice driving."

"Thanks. By the way, the old man who was APE from the shelter said thanks."

"Oh, great." He opened the second door and got a complete view of the patient. He was half on and half off the long board. The collar to keep his neck straight was around his ears The oxygen mask was on his chest and it looked like he was being strangled by the stretcher straps. But most important, he was quiet. The crew lifted out the precious cargo.

As soon as the legs of the stretcher were extended, the patient came to life. As a medic attempted to straighten him on the board, the patient raised his head and chomped down on the hand. The medic responded by slamming the patient's head forcefully backward, banging it repeatedly into the wooden long board. The patient opened his mouth fast. The other medic grabbed the patient by the throat to check for a carotid pulse.

"Are you okay?" he asked his partner.

"Yeah, it didn't break the skin."

Meanwhile the patient was turning red from the pressure applied to his neck.

"Got a pulse there, right?"

"Oh," almost forgetting himself, "yeah." As he removed his hand the patient gasped for air and became cooperative, or so it seemed. As they went to roll him, he attempted to swing and spit at the medics. He was introduced to the medic's fist and then the long board in rapid succession. Have obtained manual stabilization from his hand around the patient's throat, the medic asked his partner, "Okay, what do we do now?"

"The trauma slot." his partner said with glee.

"But . . ."

"Trust me." his partner responded.

Looking down at the cooperative patient, they rolled him into the emergency room. As they turned the corner, the lead medic yelled, "Get the trauma team, stat."

At the same time the other medic released his grip from the patient's throat. The patient had been turning blue and foaming at the mouth. His eyes looked like they would to pop out of their sockets. With the release, the patient fighting for air, started thrashing around on the stretcher.

"Look." yelled the lead medic to the eager doctors. Since it was July, most of the doctor who approached were new. The medic gave a fast report.

"High speed MVA. It was terrible. He destroyed the front end of his car by slamming into the back of a parked truck. He was okay on the scene, but as you can see his mental status is going to shit."

"Seat belt?" asked a new doctor.

"No, and the steering wheel was collapsed. He was complaining about abdominal pain."

He was rushed to the trauma slot. Going in, he attempted to bite the medic again and had his head meeting the board as well as manual stabilization applied. The doctors missed it, but the nurse looked over.

"What happened to your hand?" she asked seeing the marks on his hand, that applying manual stabilization.

"He bit me."

"Go wash that. We will take care of him," she said with a mischievous smirk on her face. The medic pushed through the onslaught of new doctors wanting to play. After washing his hands, he heard his partner call him.

"Medical consult," he said to break the discussion between his partner and a cop.

"What's up?"

"Follow me." They walked into the slot where the patient was tied down and naked.

"Doctor?" said the medic.

"Yes?"

"How's he doing?"

"He's not cooperating with us, that's for sure."

"Listen, don't forget. I told you he was grabbing his stomach on the scene."

"Oh my God," said the new doctor not wanting to miss anything, "I didn't hear that. Thank you."

The doctor grabbed his penis and a foley, a tube placed in the urinary tract and pushed until it reaches the bladder. She was not overly concerned about the size of the foley and shoved an extremely large sized one in with her right hand, as she held his penis tightly with the left. His body thrashed violently against the restraints. The medics winced through their smiles, as the screams of the patient reverberated to the waiting area.

After washing up and having a Pepsi, the crew was outside cleaning the back of the bus when one of the senior doctors approached.

"Hey. You guys didn't hit that guy busting his lip and cracking two teeth did you?"

"Us? Hell no. He was combative."

"Yeah, that's what I told him," said the doctor smiling. "Oh, by the way. Get some ice on that hand." He was now laughing.

"There is one thing I will say about you two."

"What's that?"

"You are both honest as hell."

"What?" the two medics looked puzzled.

"Ha, you really don't know do you?"

"Know what?"

"When we stripped him down he was carrying four thousand dollars cold cash on him."

"Yeah, doc we didn't know. Besides that's not our style."

"I know. You two have a style of your own." He smiled and walked inside

It was New Year's Eve in Spanish Harlem and two EMTs grabbed a fast cup of coffee, realizing they would be busy. And busy they were. Late in the evening they were called to a project on Lexington Avenue for an "unconscious."

Upon entering the location with the housing police, the officers sensed the tension. A verbal dispute erupted with several young warriors and the police.

The elevator took them to the twelfth floor, where they got off and entered the apartment. An officer was with a young male Hispanic, who sat on a couch. His mother was crying as she sat at the dining room table. Her daughter tried to console her.

The husband had died two weeks ago of a massive heart attack. The family had a modest savings. The twenty-three year old son, a drug user, was caught several times stealing his mother's jewelry and the meager food money. On several occasions, he had been physically abusive to the two women. Tonight, the combination of stealing, abuse, and drunkenness was the final straw. The mother, who spoke little English, had the nineteen-year-old daughter call 911.

As one EMT got the information, the other attempted to talk to the patient and get vital signs, blood pressure and pulse. The patient would have no part of it. He cursed the EMT and pushed his arm away. Then, in a flash, the patient jumped up, shoving past the EMT, and headed for the open window. It was dramatic, but a purely amateur act to get attention and make the mother and sister feel guilty.

The police officer and his partner lunged at him. He had only taken two steps when the EMT slammed him back onto the couch. Looking up, the EMT signaled for the handcuffs. The patient continued to struggle, as he was strapped into the stair chair and taken into the hallway.

While they waited for the elevator, the man was told to stop rocking in the chair, or it would fall over. He continued to struggle and, low and behold, it fell over. The patient's head banged into the wall and then the floor, the accompanying officers just shook their heads.

"Hey fuck this," said one EMT.

"We can't be here all night."

"Any suggestions?" asked his partner, holding the chair upright again. The patient was shouting and kicking.

"Yeah. Give him to me and open the door." With a smile on his face, he opened the hallway door to the emergency stairwell. Looking at the cops he asked, "Care to take a walk?"

"Oh, after you two gentlemen," the cops said, smiling. This stair-chaired individual went down twelve floors, bouncing all the way.

In the filthy, marijuana smoke-filled lobby, the warriors started to get out of hand. As the EMT tried to push the stair chair through the door and into the street, the patient had other ideas. With his legs extended against the door buck, he could not be moved. Shrieking at the top of his voice about police brutality and being kidnapped, he gained attention.

It started to get to critical as the pot-smoking warriors closed in and became more verbal. A riot would start if something wasn't done fast.

The EMT cursed, trying to get the patient through the door with the assistance of one officer. The other officer, hand on his drawn weapon, watched their backs.

"Fuck me," said the other EMT realizing things were about to become very bloody with the numerous warriors. He walked up to the side of the stair chair. "Excuse me," he said to the officer, who gladly stepped away.

With his back to the crowd, fearing for the safety of his partner and police officers, the EMT landed two solid blows to the patient's genital area. Needless to say, the patient closed his legs rapidly. Without missing a cue, the EMT rushed him through the door and wheeled him to the back of the bus.

"Nice style," said the EMT to his partner.

The patient was unceremoniously loaded onto the stretcher and strapped down. Off they went, with an EMT and police officer in the back and the sector car following.

Along the way, the patient made various threats. At the hospital he was rolled off of the stretcher and onto a hospital bed. He started his reign of terror against the overworked staff. At one point he cursed, then spit at the doctor and nurse tending to him.

The EMT reached to pull the dirty sheet off the stretcher, when his non-gloved hands became soaked.

"Did you piss on my stretcher?" asked the EMT.

"Yeah, fuck . . ."

Before he could finish the EMT took the urine-soaked sheet, stuffed it into the patient's mouth and squeezed. He gagged, as his urine filled his mouth, cascading down his throat.

The nurse and doctor in unison said, "Thank you."

As the EMT walked out of the room, he stopped, looked at the patient, and said in a tired voice, "No, fuck you, sir." His partner looked at him.

"What?" he asked with a smile.

"Nice style." They both laughed.

In another incident, paramedic Leonard Swade and I were told to report to CCU to be interviewed, meaning interrogated. Lenny had an idea as to why we were going and it amazed me. I complied and appeared at Puzzle Palace as directed.

Once again Steve Gilbert came to the cafeteria and said cordially, "I'll be with you shortly." He came back and said he was ready. I told him I wasn't and he'd have to wait for my attorney. He thought I was joking. He called me again and I walked in with my attorney.

"Uh, who is this?"

"This sir, is my attorney, Eileen Campbell."

"Uh, may I have your card?" he asked her, turning on the tape.

"May I have your card?" she asked. "Also, I expect a complete copy of this recording of my client."

He was in a tailspin when I walked in with her. Now he was over his head and out of his league.

What was the issue at hand? The complaint was from a nickel-and-dime security doorman in a project. It alleged, "Paramedic Leonard Swade did not give his name when asked."

He was in a tailspin when I walked in with her. Now he was over his head and out of his league.

What was the issue at hand? The complaint was from a nickel-and-dime security doorman in a project. It alleged, "Paramedic Leonard Swade did not give his name when asked."

I kid you not. We were being kept in the dark, dragged in on our day off, paid four hours overtime, to find out if one of us hadn't given our name to some below minimum wage, non-English speaking, rent-a-cop.

Even my attorney could not believe it. The whole thing was over after I stated that Joe Rent-A-Cop was interfering with our ability to treat and transport the patient.

I wasn't sure who was more in shock, Steve Gilbert, or my attorney. She was awed by the stupidity of the situation.

Kahlil Gibran, a Lebanese mystic, poet, dramatist, and artist who lived in the United States after 1910, said it best. "All work is empty save when there is love, for work is love made visible."

Some EMS crew made a lasting impression on this homeless person, considered by these students to be trash. The crew had given her a sense of dignity she would never forget. The woman's testimony spoke volumes about these EMS people, the Street Saints of Compassion.

There weren't too many girls at Club Broadway yet. Autumn had come early to the Big Apple. The brisk air coming off the river picked up speed as it moved up the concrete and steel canyon. Holding my EMS jacket closed, I hastily walked into a coffee shop. There were several Columbia University students seated around the room.

As I waited to be served, I noticed an old street woman sitting at the counter, eating her donut and drinking coffee. She wore a knee-length, gray, tattered coat, secured at the top with a safety pin. A dingy scarf hung around her neck. She appeared to be in her eighties, but looks were deceiving. Living on the streets ages people fast. Her black hair, streaked with gray, was in disarray and partially held in place by bobby pins. She was emaciated to the point that her veins stood out like straws on her dirty hands. As she lifted the donut to her thin mouth, I noticed that the dirt on part of her hands was brown, probably dry feces. She held the donut in a white napkin, contrasting sharply with her black, encrusted nails. Her eyes were sunken, as she took another bite, savoring every morsel. Behind her a wagon, loaded with bags and bottles, was covered with a filthy blanket. These were her worldly processions.

As I waited for my order, I overheard the students from Columbia snickering about the lady. She stared ahead, relishing the taste of the hot coffee. The giggles became boisterous laughter as she placed the coffee cup down. She wiped her mouth and turned to the group.

"You may think I'm filthy, uneducated, and homeless. But I am a person. And do you know who has shown me dignity and never abused me?" she asked the embarrassed intellectuals. "He has," she said pointing to me. "I am a person," she said in a stern voice turning and going back to her donut.

When I walked outside, the cool wind didn't seem to be so cold any longer. A warm feeling enveloped me as I strode, coat open, back to the unit. I had witnessed a sacred blessing. Somewhere along the way, one of our crewmembers, wearing the same green jacket, pants, and white shirt, had shown this woman respect.

The Dance of Life was a beautiful thing when we had people like Bryan, Alex, and John on our team. It was even more pleasurable when we had a team effort, like Rescue One helping at one end and Bellevue Hospital at the other.

Bouncing along, Bryan got two 14 gauge catheters into the patient's arms as he continued to assess his condition. Soon we pulled into the bay of the hospital.

As we offloaded and made our way into the "slot," a special room for trauma patients, the staff was ready. The dance continued. The system had worked for one soul.

One person we all learned to know and hate was a man we labeled 32X, better known as Wilbur Zachary. This individual always called for a bus, claiming to be a quadriplegic. He purported to have a lawsuit against every hospital in Manhattan. I first met him years before as an EMT.

We received a call for an "Injury." Pulling up, my seasoned partner recognized 32X right away. Before getting out of the vehicle, he asked me if I knew the patient.

"No," I replied.

"Okay, watch and learn."

Getting out, we approached the patient, sitting on a stoop in Spanish Harlem. The street glistened from the rain that had fallen earlier in the evening.

"Hey, Zach, what's up?"

"I need to go to the hospital."

"Okay. Get in the ambulance and let's go."

"I can't. I'm a quad and you'll have to carry me. That's your job." My partner looked at me then to 32X.

"How did you get here?" No answer. "Okay, asshole. Let's go." With this, 32X was grabbed under both arms and assisted to the unit where he *stepped up* into the vehicle.

"I'm going for a soda," I said, "do you want anything?" "No thanks. You go and I'll get the vitals."

"Yeah, I want a beer," 32X said.

"Whatever," I responded, heading across the rain-slicked street to the bodega. "Ready?" I asked upon returning.

"Yeah," my partner responded, "let's go to Metropolitan Hospital."

As the back door was being closed, 32X asked, "Hey! Where's my beer?"

"It wasn't cold yet," I said, closing the door. At the hospital, I came to the back to find the quadriplegic standing on the rear bumper.

"Hey, don't stand there," my partner warned. "He just pissed on the rear bumper and emergency bay ramp."

"You did what?" I uttered in disbelief.

"Yeah, I did! Want me to piss on you?" 32X yelled, as he reached for his zipper. There was one tremendous bang as 32X *slipped* and *crashed* onto the floor of the unit. Hey trust me, it happens. Then grabbing 32X by his collar and belt, I dragged him off the unit as my partner grabbed the other side. We approached the automatic doors on the emergency bay ramp, which were slow in opening. Zach was still screaming, cursing, and threatening to sue us. The darn doors' timing was off, as poor 32X's head became a battering ram till they opened.

Before getting to the second set of doors, my partner said, "We can't bring him in like this. I'll get a chair," instantly releasing Zach's squirming, thrashing body.

32X continued his tirade of screaming, threats and curses. I, now alone and holding him, said, "No I'll get a chair." Hey, wheelchairs are hard to find.

In a sudden flash of realization he looked up at me. There came a final loud scream, as I smiled, then silence, as 32X crashed to the floor. Once we got the chair, 32X played the "I can't move" routine. So we hoisted then dumped the quadriplegic into the chair. As the strap went across his chest, he came to life, shrieking he did not want to be strapped in. A seat belt is a good thing. As he was rolled into the emergency room, everyone looked, realized who it was, then went back to work. Trying to get him into the triage area was a problem, since the "quad" was kicking, flailing his legs, arms and cursing. A black female Hop Cop attempted to help and talk Wilbur.

"Fuck you. You can suck my dick, you black nigger bi—" Before he could continue, I accidentally ran the patient into the closed door, catapulting him and sending him crashing to the floor. "Remember what I said about seat belt safety?" I asked, picking him up and dumping Zach back in the chair. The officer quickly opened the door and Wilbur was pushed into the area. Sitting between the officer and me, 32X started screaming.

"Do you always treat black people like this?"

Reaching into my pocket, I asked, "Can you read?"

"Sure I can read." He responded indignantly.

"What does this say?"

"NAACP."

"Correct, Wilbur. NAACP. This means that I support black people. It also means that I do not treat blacks any different than anyone else. It does mean that I treat niggers all the same, no matter what color they are. Now this officer is black and is my friend, so show some respect, nigger."

The officer nodded her agreement, looking at a stunned 32X, "What are you looking at, nigger?" Yes, I did indeed have a NAACP card and was a paid, proud member. I found it worked wonders in shutting up loud-mouth blacks as they hid behind their race, the same way EMS supervision hid behind rank, and chiefs hid behind charge packages. Bottom line is we are all one.

Wilbur did make a complaint to EMS, and, of course, all panicked. That was until the statement went in with the Hop Cop's statement and my NAACP card number. Another word was never heard.

The same cannot be said about Wilbur. Through the years he continued to plague the units, sometimes calling in false 10-13s ("Cop Shot") to get attention. One night, a Basic crew got him. They'd had a rough evening and were not in the mood as they lifted the uncooperative *patient* onto the stretcher. Once in the back of the bus, they slammed the doors, rolling him on his stomach. His eyes darted, as they took off their equipment belts and started to unzip their pants.

Panicking, he yelled, rolling over, "What are you doing?"

"We've had it with you, asshole. So now we are going to fuck you in the ass."

"Oh God, please, no!" he begged, curling into a ball, using his arms and legs which a minute ago didn't work. The day before, he almost had the same crew hurt by inciting the locals who thought the crew didn't want to do their job and carry the "hurt man." Tonight, they were seething.

"Roll over, motherfucker!" One EMT screamed, grabbing for 32X's belt and zipper. Pulling his pants and shorts down was easy as they rolled him onto his stomach, as he continued to wail. The radio traffic was constant, as the one EMT looked at the other and smiled.

"Hey! Strap this piece of shit in. I know where we'll take him."

They strapped him face down, ass in the air, on the stretcher. The EMT floored it, only stopping after they entered the infamous Hunts Point Fish Market, South Bronx. They had left Manhattan, went deep into the South Bronx, all with no radio signal. Once there, they dragged the hysterical, pleading 32X out of the vehicle.

"On your knees, asshole!" With his pants and shorts still down around his ankles they placed a mini mag flashlight behind his ear.

"We are sick of you in Manhattan, motherfucker. Tonight I'm going to kill you once and for all."

The tears rolled down 32X's face. He blubbered like a baby. The crew had positioned him so he was kneeling in a puddle of fish and diesel-polluted water.

"Down!" screamed one EMT, trying not to laugh. "On your chest, motherfucker!" his partner commanded in a now unemotional voice. The grim, demonic, lifeless voice petrified Zach. Now truly paralyzed for the first time in his life, he left a faint whimper escape his lips as he fell forward into the putrid puddle of cold water. Thus 32X was face down in the water, his bare ass to the sky with what he perceived as a small-caliber gun to his head. The radio went off. "We haven't got time to finish him now," said the one EMT. "Let's do the next job and come back for the shithead." The one with the *weapon* roughly grabbed 32X by his collar. "Don't move. We'll be back." He hissed. With this, they drove off into the night, hysterical.

I was working overtime on a medic unit the next day. I had heard the story that circulated the garage. Finally, this crew had outdone all others concerning 32X. In the office were Lieutenant Barrios, two chiefs, and an ISU on unrelated business. However, as I sat there reading, an article jumped out of the paper: "Male black found dead in Hunt's Point fish market." At that moment, the crew came walking through the door. I looked at them then the article. This was too priceless to pass up. They froze as they saw all the brass in the other office.

"Hey, guys. You made the paper. Nice going," I said, showing them the article. Sheer panic set in, as they begged me not to say a word and get rid of the article. I looked at them, both good guys. "Okay," I said, taking the page out and stuffing it in my shirt. No one ever saw or heard from 32X again. Hey, coincidences happen, yeah right . . . trust me!

Also By Jim Schrang

Civilian Warriors, Civilian Healers

And

Alicia 'Unworthy Life'

Made in the USA
Monee, IL
08 November 2026

67970056R00157